# Culturally Informed Therapy for Schizophrenia

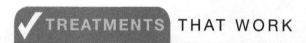
# TREATMENTS THAT WORK

**Editor-In-Chief**

David H. Barlow, PhD

**Scientific Advisory Board**

Anne Marie Albano, PhD

Gillian Butler, PhD

David M. Clark, PhD

Edna B. Foa, PhD

Paul J. Frick, PhD

Jack M. Gorman, MD

Kirk Heilbrun, PhD

Robert J. McMahon, PhD

Peter E. Nathan, PhD

Christine Maguth Nezu, PhD

Matthew K. Nock, PhD

Paul Salkovskis, PhD

Bonnie Spring, PhD

Gail Steketee, PhD

John R. Weisz, PhD

G. Terence Wilson, PhD

# Culturally Informed Therapy for Schizophrenia

A Family-Focused Cognitive Behavioral Approach

**CLINICIAN GUIDE**

AMY WEISMAN DE MAMANI

MERRANDA MCLAUGHLIN

OLIVIA ALTAMIRANO

DAISY LOPEZ

SALMAN SHAHEEN AHMAD

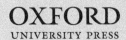

OXFORD
UNIVERSITY PRESS

# OXFORD
UNIVERSITY PRESS

Oxford University Press is a department of the University of Oxford. It furthers
the University's objective of excellence in research, scholarship, and education
by publishing worldwide. Oxford is a registered trade mark of Oxford University
Press in the UK and certain other countries.

Published in the United States of America by Oxford University Press
198 Madison Avenue, New York, NY 10016, United States of America.

Library of Congress Cataloging-in-Publication Data
Names: Weisman de Mamani, Amy, author.
Title: Culturally informed therapy for schizophrenia : a family-focused
cognitive behavioral approach, clinician guide / Amy Weisman de Mamani,
Merranda McLaughlin, Olivia Altamirano, Daisy Lopez, Salman Shaheen Ahmad.
Description: New York, NY : Oxford University Press, [2021] |
Series: Treatments that work | Includes bibliographical references and index.
Identifiers: LCCN 2020026336 (print) | LCCN 2020026337 (ebook) |
ISBN 9780197500644 (paperback) | ISBN 9780197500668 (epub) |
ISBN 9780197500675
Subjects: LCSH: Schizophrenia—Treatment. | Evidence-based medicine. |
Family therapy. | Cultural psychiatry.
Classification: LCC RC514 .W418 2021 (print) | LCC RC514 (ebook) |
DDC 616.89/8—dc23
LC record available at https://lccn.loc.gov/2020026336
LC ebook record available at https://lccn.loc.gov/2020026337

9 8 7 6 5 4 3 2 1

Printed by Marquis, Canada

I dedicate this book to Giovanni, my precious son. Thanks for your understanding and patience while I spent many weekend and evening hours away from home, working on this book. I love you!

—Amy Weisman de Mamani

I dedicate this book to the mentors who have paved the way for me to be here, but especially to the original two, my mom and dad. Your love and influence have shaped me in ways I hope to continue to uncover.

—Merranda McLaughlin

To Mom and Dad

—Salman Shaheen Ahmad

Stunning developments in healthcare have taken place over the last several years, but many of our widely accepted interventions and strategies in mental health and behavioral medicine have been brought into question by research evidence as not only lacking benefit, but perhaps, inducing harm (Barlow, 2010). Other strategies have been proven effective using the best current standards of evidence, resulting in broad-based recommendations to make these practices more available to the public (McHugh & Barlow, 2010). Several recent developments are behind this revolution. First, we have arrived at a much deeper understanding of pathology, both psychological and physical, which has led to the development of new, more precisely targeted interventions. Second, our research methodologies have improved substantially, such that we have reduced threats to internal and external validity, making the outcomes more directly applicable to clinical situations. Third, governments around the world and healthcare systems and policymakers have decided that the quality of care should improve, that it should be evidence based, and that it is in the public's interest to ensure that this happens (Barlow, 2004; Institute of Medicine, 2001, 2015; McHugh & Barlow, 2010).

Of course, the major stumbling block for clinicians everywhere is the accessibility of newly developed evidence-based psychological interventions. Workshops and books can go only so far in acquainting responsible and conscientious practitioners with the latest behavioral healthcare practices and their applicability to individual patients. This series, Treatments *ThatWork*™, is devoted to communicating these exciting new interventions to clinicians on the frontlines of practice.

The manuals and workbooks in this series contain step-by-step detailed procedures for assessing and treating specific problems and diagnoses. But this series also goes beyond the books and manuals by providing ancillary materials that will approximate the supervisory process in assisting practitioners in the implementation of these procedures in their practice.

In our emerging healthcare system, the growing consensus is that evidence-based practice offers the most responsible course of action for the mental health professional. All behavioral healthcare clinicians deeply desire to provide the best possible care for their patients. In this series, our aim is to close the dissemination and information gap and make that possible.

This guide addresses the treatment of schizophrenia with a 15-week family therapy protocol that is designed to be implemented in an outpatient mental health setting. It is estimated that approximately 1 in 100 adults in the United States will be diagnosed with schizophrenia or a related schizophrenia spectrum disorder. The guide is intended to be used by clinicians who are already familiar with cognitive-behavioral therapy generally and have some background in treating serious mental illness. Because the processes and techniques that are presented here build upon treatment protocols with extensive empirical support accumulated over several decades, *Culturally Informed Therapy for Schizophrenia: A Family-Focused Cognitive Behavioral Approach, Clinician Guide* will be an indispensable resource for all practitioners who wish to effectively and efficiently help individuals with schizophrenia reduce their symptoms and assist them and their loved ones to improve the quality of their lives.

David H. Barlow, Editor-in-Chief
Treatments *That Work*™
Boston, Massachusetts

# Contents

Foreword    *xi*

Acknowledgments    *xiii*

Chapter 1       Introduction    *1*

Chapter 2       Background and CIT-S Overview    *9*

Chapter 3       Module 1—Family Collectivism
                (Sessions 1–3)    *23*

Chapter 4       Module 2—Psychoeducation
                (Sessions 4–6)    *35*

Chapter 5       Module 3—Spirituality (Sessions 7–9)    *51*

Chapter 6       Module 4—Communication Training
                (Sessions 10–12)    *67*

Chapter 7       Module 5—Problem-Solving
                (Sessions 13–15)    *87*

Chapter 8       Additional Considerations    *103*

Chapter 9       Integrated CIT-S Illustration    *111*

Appendix: Handouts    *137*
References    *161*

Individuals living with schizophrenia spectrum disorders confront many challenges—distressing beliefs and experiences; cognitive impairments in executive planning, memory, attention, and concentration; and problems with motivation, socialization, and the expression of a range of affect. Medications can address some of these issues, but they rarely result alone in a full return to satisfactory functioning. Rather, engagement in psychosocial interventions in combination with taking prescribed medications typically result in the best outcomes.

Family therapy is a psychosocial intervention grounded in 40 years of research supporting its use in schizophrenia spectrum disorders. Participation in family therapies, which include specific core features (illness education, communication skills training, problem-solving instruction, directive and structured sessions, and de-emphasis on psychodynamic interpretations), can galvanize social support for recovery and reduce relapse rates in schizophrenia by 30% to 50%. Engagement in family therapy programs is also linked to improved well-being of relatives of the individuals living with schizophrenia.

In this text, Weisman de Mamani and colleagues bring a fresh eye to family therapy for schizophrenia, informed by their 20 years of research in this area; they provide an accessible, easy-to-use clinician guide to support the recovery of individuals living with schizophrenia spectrum disorders. Equally important, these authors have found a way to address one of the most vexing problems in this field: How can mental health providers implement a manualized evidence-based intervention while still tailoring it to the unique cultural needs of the participants? Weisman de Mamani and colleagues have found an innovative strategy to integrate attention to cultural norms and complex issues such as spirituality and religion with the core components of evidence-based family therapy; their preliminary data reflect the benefits of using this more holistic intervention. Their approach is novel, useable, respectful, and compassionate.

This book provides a hands-on introduction to culturally informed therapy for schizophrenia (CIT-S), replete with an informative, intellectually compelling introductory chapter on cultural issues in mental health treatment, as well as interesting case examples and well-designed handouts. As more and more societies become multicultural, there is an increasing expectation that mental health providers will meet the needs of unique populations in an efficient, skillful, yet caring manner. While recognition of diversity is now a cornerstone of most graduate programs, most providers continue to require ongoing training and support throughout their careers to optimize outcomes of the many cultural groups presenting for their care. *Culturally Informed Therapy for Schizophrenia: A Family-Focused Cognitive Behavioral Approach, Clinician Guide* helps fill that gap and is a wonderful resource for mental health practitioners working with individuals living with schizophrenia spectrum disorders and their loved ones.

Shirley M. Glynn, PhD
Research Psychologist
Semel Institute of Neuroscience
and Human Behavior, UCLA

# Acknowledgments

The first author of this book, Amy Weisman de Mamani, PhD, expresses gratitude to the many people who have contributed to the development and evaluation of CIT-S. First and foremost, I would like to acknowledge the hundreds of individuals with schizophrenia and their family members who have participated in our intervention studies and have greatly helped us to evaluate and refine our treatment. I have been inspired by so many of you for the richness of your lives and for your willingness and dedication to love one another and to work together as a family. I also want to thank my mentors Margaret Rae, Shirley Glynn, and especially the late Michael Goldstein who introduced me to family therapy for serious mental illness and supervised my early training in this area. You instilled in me a sense of passion for and a lifelong interest in this line of work. I am also indebted to David Miklowitz, Harriet Lefley, Ian Falloon, and countless others whose body of work has greatly inspired and shaped my own thinking and research path. Additionally, thanks go to the numerous graduate students and research assistants over the years, who served as clinicians, assessors, translators, data analysts, and editors of my manuscripts on CIT-S. Without you all, this book could never have come to fruition. Finally, I thank Kate Scheinman, my fabulous developmental editor, whose very thoughtful feedback has greatly enhanced the organization and quality of this book!

# CHAPTER 1

# Introduction

## Purpose of This Book

This book describes culturally informed therapy for schizophrenia (CIT-S), a 15-week, family-based intervention for treating individuals with schizophrenia spectrum disorders (SSD) and their family members. It provides the theoretical background for CIT-S and a step-by-step guide to conducting the intervention. While several psychotherapies for schizophrenia exist (e.g., Roberts, Penn, & Combs, 2015), few systematically incorporate clients' cultural beliefs, values, and practices into the intervention. Thus, these interventions may be less relevant for individuals from certain ethnic and cultural backgrounds. Additionally, existing interventions do not systematically incorporate family members and others closest to those coping with an SSD into treatment, despite the fact that there is evidence that schizophrenia is highly responsive to the emotional atmosphere of the family. Research suggests that sociocultural factors play a central role in adjustment to this disorder for both people with an SSD and their family members (Lefley, 1990; Weisman, Gurak, & Suro, 2014). By treating the client in isolation, without their loved ones, prior interventions may have a more limited impact on the sociocultural environment in which a person resides and operates.

## Who Is This Book For?

This intervention is most relevant for clinicians and researchers interested in treating individuals with SSDs and their close family members.

*Clinician Note*

*One word of caution is that clients who are currently in the midst of an acute psychotic episode do not make good candidates for CIT-S. The rationale for this perception is discussed in more detail in Chapter 8, where we suggest that such clients should first be referred out for medication management and then encouraged to return once stabilized. In Chapter 8, we also offer guidance on how to determine if a client is currently displaying levels of psychosis too high to benefit from treatment.*

We define family broadly and refer to genetic kin, romantic partners, and any other close friends who have a long-term commitment to the care of an individual with schizophrenia. While the treatment is specifically developed for individuals with SSD, it is important to point out that improving the lives of family members who care for (and about) individuals with SSDs is also an important and *direct* goal of CIT-S. This is different from many other family treatments that include family members in therapy primarily to the extent that they can aid in the recovery of the person with mental illness.

Thus, if you are a mental health treatment provider who works with clients with SSDs, this book may be for you. If you are a person with an SSD or a family member of one, you may also benefit from this book as a form of self-help or as an accompaniment to another psychotherapy approach. As the treatment draws heavily from clients' own cultural, religious, and spiritual beliefs, values, and traditions, CIT-S is relevant for individuals from any race and ethnic or cultural group. There is no intention to "teach" clients about cultural and religious factors. Rather, the aim is to have clients educate clinicians about their own cultural and religious beliefs, practices, and traditions. Clinicians then utilize this information to help guide clients to create healthy and harmonious environments that are in line with their values and that, ultimately, will allow them to better manage mental illness and improve the quality of their lives.

## Credentials Required to Deliver CIT-S

In our view, clinicians who deliver CIT-S should be licensed mental health practitioners (e.g., psychologists, MSWs), or doctoral students or master's level students in supervision with a licensed practitioner who is qualified to deliver CIT-S. As CIT-S draws largely from a cognitive behavioral framework (e.g., Sokol & Fox, 2019), some background in this orientation is necessary. Finally, as CIT-S is a family-focused intervention, clinicians should have received some prior training in family-oriented and systems approaches (e.g., Conoley & Conoley, 2009; Lebow, 2015) or should receive supervision from someone who has the appropriate training.

## Organization of the Book

In Chapter 1, we have thus far described the purpose of the book and discussed who it is intended to serve. The remainder of this chapter will outline the organization of the book. In Chapter 2, we describe the signs and symptoms of SSDs and provide the theoretical rationale behind CIT-S. Next, we provide an overview of CIT-S and describe the empirical literature supporting the efficacy of the intervention. In Chapters 3 to 7, we offer an in-depth, session-by-session guide for implementing each of the five modules of the intervention. Each module is accompanied by detailed handouts to guide that treatment segment, suggested homework assignments, and a case example to illustrate how the module can be applied to individuals from diverse ethnic and cultural backgrounds. The cases capture common familial structures including nuclear families, single-parent households, same-sex couples, and mixed-race couples. They also encompass a range of religious orientations such as Christianity, Islam, Judaism, and atheism. It is important to note here that these case illustrations are fictional. While many of the events, stories, and issues that are depicted in these cases are drawn from our experiences with actual clients in CIT-S, we have altered their names, demographics, and storylines to make sure that no client is recognizable.

In Chapter 8, we discuss working with clients who are unmedicated and displaying high levels of psychosis. We also discuss issues around whether it is important for clinicians and clients to be similar in ethnicity and other cultural beliefs and values, and we offer suggestions for dealing with challenging clients and families. Finally, in Chapter 9, we provide an integrated hypothetical case example of CIT-S that illustrates each module within a single family.

It is important to clarify how we are defining certain words and terms in this book. For race and ethnicity in particular, we attempted to use terms that are (a) inclusive of all individuals we are aiming to include in the definition and ideally (b) used by the group we are referencing. However, regardless of the term used, we are endeavoring to describe heterogeneous groups of people, some of whom may prefer alternative terms. In addition, concepts of race and ethnicity shift over time, so while we attempt to use appropriate terminology in this book, we recognize current and future readers may prefer different labels.

In this book, we use the label *H/L* to define people who identify as Hispanic, Latino/a, or Latinx. The term *Hispanic* comes from the Latin word *Hispania*, which later became *España* (Spain) and refers to people who are from countries where the primary language is Spanish (Salinas, 2015). This term was first adopted by the U.S. government during Richard Nixon's presidency and was implemented in the U.S. Census in 1980 (Delgado-Romero, Manlove, Manlove, & Hernandez, 2006). The term *Latino* was adapted by the U.S. government to refer to people from Mexico and the Caribbean and the countries that comprise Central and South America, including those that are not Spanish-speaking such as Belize, Brazil, French Guiana, Guyana, and Suriname (De Luca & Escoto, 2012). *Latino* also refers to people who identify as mestizo or mulatto (mixed White, with Black and Native) people of Central or South America (Delgado-Romero et al., 2006). The term *Latinx* emerged much more recently as a gender-inclusive replacement for *Latino/a* (Salinas & Lozano, 2017). While there are certainly many subgroup differences among individuals under the H/L umbrella, they also share many commonalities including a tendency toward a more collectivistic self-construal, a strong emphasis placed on the family, and religious sensibilities that shape and give meaning to their lives (Suarez-Orozco & Páez, 2002; Telzer et al., 2010; Turcios-Cotto & Milan, 2013). Studies suggest that H/Ls, relative to other ethnic groups, tend to remain loyal to their native language and the majority, even those living in the United States, have some proficiency in and a strong connection to the Spanish language (Suarez-Orozco & Páez, 2002; Mora, Villa, & Dávila, 2006; Alba, Logan, Lutz, & Stults, 2002).

We use the term *Asian* to refer to a broad group of individuals who have origins in East Asia, South Asia, or Southeast Asia, as defined by the U.S. Census Bureau (Humes, Jones, & Ramirez, 2011). Among Asian people, the family unit tends to be highly prized and emphasized throughout the life cycle more so than in White families, in which parents and other members of the nuclear family are more likely to encourage and value independence, autonomy, and self-sufficiency of individual members of the nuclear family, especially as they reach adulthood (Lee & Mock, 2005). Common Asian values, which may be highly relevant to consider in therapy with this group, include self-control, suppression of emotion, and a short-term, result-oriented solution to problems (Lee & Mock, 2005).

We use the term *White* to refer to people who are of European descent who do not identify as H/L, although at times this term is also used to refer to Americans of North African and Middle Eastern descent (U.S. Census Bureau, 2011). White people in the United States have been the most resistant to ethnic labels (Giordano & McGoldrick, 2005; McDermott & Samson, 2005). However, research shows that this group of individuals does share some commonalities, including a belief system that views time as a commodity, a view of the individual as the primary unit of society, and a notion that status is best measured by credentials, possessions, titles, and professions (Giordano & McGoldrick, 2005; Lincoln, Chatters, & Taylor, 2003; Zha, Walczyk, Griffith-Ross, Tobacyk, & Walczyk, 2006).

We use the term *Black* to refer to individuals who have ancestry in any of the Black racial groups of Africa (U.S. Census Bureau, 2011). While the term *African American* is also used within the United States, it is often used in reference to Black Americans descendant from people who were brought to the Americas and enslaved from the 17th to 19th century (Agyemang, Bhopal, & Bruijnzeels, 2005). This may exclude African Caribbean/Black Caribbean individuals, which refers to people with African ancestry who migrated to the Caribbean. Although *Black* refers to a very heterogeneous collection of people, as a group, religion and spirituality have been particularly important factors in the lives of Black people living in the United States, with three out of every four reporting that religion is *extremely* important in their day to day functioning (Black & Jackson, 2005). Family structures often tend to be extended with three or more generations living in a home, and the role of the grandmother is often central in Black American families (Hines & Boyd-Franklin, 2005). Hines and Boyd-Franklin (2005) argue that Black individuals have very strong kinship bonds that are traceable to Africa, where various tribes shared commonalities that were stronger than bloodlines. They further contend that because Black people had the worldview that they owed their existence to the tribe, even today Black people often hold the collectivistic philosophy of "we are; therefore, I am" as opposed to the more individualistic focus from a mainstream, White U.S. perspective (Nobles, 2004). We use the terms *White* and *Black* rather than alternatives (such as *Euro American* or *African American*) because these terms are less tied to specific countries/continents than their alternatives.

It is also important to point out that, in this book, we generally do not add the descriptor *American* (e.g., Asian American) for any ethnic group, unless we are reporting results of a specific study (e.g., Mexican Americans). This is because, despite the fact that this book is generally intended for clients and clinicians living in the United States and many clients may be United States citizens or permanent residents, others may be visiting, reside abroad for part of the year, or simply do not identify as American. Thus, the term *American* does not add specificity and in some cases may be inaccurate; therefore, we chose not to include it.

It is important to note that we view race and ethnicity as primarily social constructs, as opposed to predominantly biological indicators. In this vein, we consider our client's sense of their own race/ethnicity as much more salient in treatment than other genotypic or phenotypic characteristics (such as what they look like). Thus, in our research studies, clients' ethnicity/race is often designated based on their own self-report of these constructs.

In the same vein, clinicians should ensure they also ask clients about their gender identity and use the pronouns that the individual endorses. Importantly, clinicians should avoid making assumptions; an individual may identify as nonbinary, but prefer he/him/his or she/her/hers pronouns or have undergone surgery to present as masculine/feminine but prefer they/them/theirs pronouns. In this book, we frequently use *they* as a singular, gender-neutral pronoun. For the purpose of our case illustrations, we have utilized she/her/hers and he/him/his pronouns as, to date, all of our clients in CIT-S endorsed these pronouns and have identified as cisgender. However, we believe the goals of CIT-S are in line with working with a multitude of identities and cultures, and we hope subsequent iterations of this clinician guide may provide additional insights that may prove beneficial to clinicians and their clients with these and/or other identities.

We use the word *minority* to refer to people of limited power and disadvantage rather than referring to the size of the group relative to others. This is because certain groups such as H/Ls are expected to surpass non-H/L White individuals by the middle of the century (and already have in some cohorts, such as generation Z; Passel, Livingston, & Cohn, 2012) yet are still disadvantaged in terms of economic and political power (De Jong & Madamba, 2001; Kempf-Leonard, 2007). Similarly, women outnumber men in the United States and much of the rest of the world, yet financially, professionally, and in other ways (e.g., holding powerful political positions) still fare more poorly than their male counterparts (Le & Miller, 2010; Lawless & Pearson, 2008).

When we discuss religious groups (e.g., Muslims, Christians, Jews), we are generally referring to a group of individuals who may be from any ethnic-cultural or racial background. Of course, this line is sometimes blurred. For example, Jewish identity has been historically grounded in both genealogical and religious heritage (Glenn, 2002), and to the extent a Jewish individual identifies with one or both of those aspects can influence their sense of self (Friedman, Friedlander, & Blustein, 2005; Hecht & Faulkner, 2000; Weisskirch, Kim, Schwartz, & Whitbourne, 2016).

With respect to the terms *religion* and *spirituality*, we generally use the term *religion* to refer to specific creeds, rituals, sacraments, etc. that are associated with an identifiable faith. On the other hand, the term *spirituality* will be used more often to refer to one's quest for meaning and belonging and to the core values that influence one's behavior, which are not necessarily tied to a specific doctrine or canon. Occasionally, we use the abbreviation *R/S* when it is difficult to separate the concepts, as some scholars argue that they cannot be unlinked. Zinnbauer and Pargament (2005), for example, place spirituality within the broader construct of religion. They suggest that spirituality serves as the core of religion, with religion referring to a broader range of behaviors than does the term spirituality. Koenig (2012) similarly argues that spirituality is an exten-sion of religion, where those who report themselves to be at the highest levels of religion are considered spiritual. In this book, therefore, when we are making no distinction, we will use the abbreviation *R/S*, but will continue to separate the terms otherwise, as previously described.

Finally, we use the word *intersectionality* to refer to the interconnected nature of social categorizations such as race, class, and gender as they apply to a given individual or group. Overlapping and interdependent identities can lead to more complex forms of discrimination and dis-advantage in some cases. Having multiple identities can also impart unique and compounded strengths, as people have a greater number of experiences, value systems, and often resources to draw from, which can assist them in managing mental illness and other adversities.

# CHAPTER 2

# Background and CIT-S Overview

## Background Information

Schizophrenia is a severe mental disorder, affecting approximately 1% to 4% of the population worldwide (Saha, Chant, Welham, & McGrath, 2005; Bhugra, 2005). Primary symptoms of this disorder include hallucinations, delusions, thought disorder, negative symptoms (amotivation, anhedonia, flat affect), and grossly disorganized or catatonic behavior, with cognitive decline being common prior to and during onset of the illness (Tandon et al., 2013).

Research clearly indicates biological underpinnings for the disorder (e.g., Walker, Kestler, Bollini, & Hochman, 2004), and there is evidence from many clinical trials that antipsychotic medications are effective in reducing acute symptoms (Bradford, Stroup, & Liberman, 2002). There is now mounting evidence that schizophrenia is also highly responsive to the emotional atmosphere of the family. Research suggests that sociocultural factors play a central role in both patients' and family members' adjustment to this disorder (Lefley, 1990; Weisman, Gurak, & Suro, 2014). Moreover, existing family-oriented psychoeducational interventions for schizophrenia, combined with antipsychotic medication, have been found to be effective in reducing or delaying relapse and rehospitalization (Lucksted, McFarlane, Downing, & Dixon, 2012). However, few existing programs are culturally informed and may be less relatable and relevant for many minority groups, including Black and Hispanic, Latino/a, or Latinx (H/L) families, who overwhelmingly report turning to spiritual and allocentric values when coping with mental illness (Caqueo-Urizar, Urzúa, Boyer, & Williams, 2016; Black & Jackson, 2005; Chatters, Taylor, Jackson, & Lincoln, 2008; Mohr et al., 2012). Attention to these values does not appear to be a major focus of most existing empirically based family treatments for schizophrenia, although many minorities report benefits from coping through these mechanisms.

## Culture and the Environment

Expressed emotion (EE), a measure of critical, hostile, and emotionally overinvolved attitudes (e.g., intrusiveness, self-sacrificing behaviors) from a family member toward a person with mental illness, has been found to be a robust predictor of symptom relapse among those with psychosis (Weintraub, Hall, Carbonella, Weisman de Mamani, & Hooley, 2016; O'Driscoll, Sener, Angmark, & Shaikh, 2019). Despite this and the approximately equivalent prevalence rates of schizophrenia worldwide, international research in psychopathology indicates that empathy and support patterns toward relatives with mental illness vary dramatically across national and ethnic groups (Lopez et al., 2009). In general, relatives of individuals from developing or traditional cultures (i.e., societies that are collectivistic and tradition-oriented) tend to be less critical than their more industrialized counterparts (Singh, Harley, & Suhail, 2013). For example, White family members in London tend to have greater rates of high EE compared to family members in India (Singh et al., 2013). This variability has even been observed within the United States. For example, the prevalence of high EE in families in the Los Angeles area was three times greater in White families than in H/L families of Mexican descent (Jenkins, Karno, de la Selva, & Santana, 1986). Telles and colleagues (1995) also found cultural differences in EE patterns. In this study, only 7% of families of recent Salvadoran, Honduran, and Mexican immigrants were rated as highly critical, whereas earlier research indicates the rate is 10 times higher for White families living in the same geographic area. In fact, Weisman de Mamani and colleagues (2007) found that White family members of people with schizophrenia in Boston, Los Angeles, and Miami were rated as exhibiting over three times greater rates of high EE as compared to H/L caregivers.

People from different cultures may also experience EE differently. For example, Rosenfarb, Bellack, and Aziz (2006) found that, among Black individuals, greater perceived criticism was associated with better outcomes such as decreased unusual thinking over a two-year period. Gurak and Weisman de Mamani (2017) corroborated these results, finding greater symptom severity among Black individuals with a low EE caregiver. It has been argued that communication patterns among Black individuals are livelier (Rogan & Hammer, 1998), and many comments and expressions that are viewed as critical from a White person's perspective may not be viewed as such from a Black person's perspective. This may suggest that measurements of EE may be limited and not generalizable to all groups. Interestingly, Weisman, Rosales, Kymalainen, and Armesto (2006) offer some empirical evidence that the perceptions of people with schizophrenia spectrum disorders (SSDs) of their relatives' criticism may differ by ethnicity. As predicted, Weisman et al. (2006) found that White and H/L family members who were designated as expressing more criticism by researchers during an EE interview were indeed perceived as more critical by their relative with schizophrenia. Among Black participants, however, they did not find an association between relatives' expressed criticism and the perception of people with SSDs of their relatives' criticism. These findings highlight the different roles EE can play in different cultural contexts. They also underscore the need to assess perceived EE of family members from the perspective of the person coping with mental illness.

Differences in the prevalence of high EE appear to form a cultural pattern in terms of schizophrenia relapse rates. The International Pilot study of Schizophrenia suggests that patients from the developing nations of Nigeria, India, and Colombia had a more favorable course than patients from industrialized countries such as Denmark, the former Czechoslovakia, the United Kingdom, the former USSR, and the United States (Jablensky et al., 1992). Additionally, Wüsten and Lincoln (2017) found that individuals from developing countries, as compared to those from industrialized countries, perceive more support and are more satisfied with their relationships. Thus, although schizophrenia appears to occur cross-culturally, the course of the disorder and family members' reactions to it seem to be significantly influenced by sociocultural forces.

The different percentages of high EE families between Mexican Americans and White Americans living in the United States seems to parallel qualitative data regarding the attributions the two groups make for their relative's disorder. Jenkins et al. (1986) noted that high EE Mexican Americans appear less accepting of the illness-based view of the disorder than were low EE Mexican Americans. On the whole, however, Mexican Americans were much more likely to view the problem as one of illness than were White individuals who were more likely to attribute it to personality characteristics, irrespective of EE status. Jenkins (1986) found that Mexican American key relatives were far less likely to criticize symptom behaviors than were their White counterparts. In addition, Mexican Americans often associated the illness with one's nervous or mental condition or some other biological problem. The authors noted that belief in the legitimacy of schizophrenia as an illness was linked to views that symptom behaviors generally lie outside the patient's personal control.

In addition to marked qualitative differences in attitudes regarding schizophrenia, Jenkins et al. (1986) also reported qualitative differences in the emotional reactions to the disorder between Mexican Americans and White individuals living in the United States. For Mexican Americans, the most common emotional reactions toward the illness were sadness, sorrow, and pity. While White individuals also reported feelings of sadness (especially those low in EE), these were less frequent than other negative emotions such as anger and annoyance. Mexican American verbalizations of sadness were also frequently accompanied by evidence of warmth and sympathy for the person with mental illness and their condition. Mexican Americans also showed more tolerance, patience, and respect toward the person with schizophrenia. In fact, Lopez and colleagues (2004) found that warmth served as a protective factor against relapse among Mexican Americans with schizophrenia, but family criticism was a significant risk factor for relapse among White Americans. Therefore, not only are there differences in emotional responses to schizophrenia among cultural groups, but these distinctions may play a significant role in the illness' trajectory in different ways.

Weisman and López (1997) directly tested for cultural differences between Mexicans residing in Mexico and White Americans living in the United States. In this study, Mexicans were much more external in perceptions of control and less blaming in their attributions about schizophrenia than were White Americans. White Americans also reported feeling more intense unfavorable emotions toward the person with schizophrenia.

The previously reviewed research suggests that cultural differences observed in family members' reactions to schizophrenia may shed light on the puzzling observation by the World Health Organization. As reviewed earlier, their multisite international pilot study (Jablensky et al., 1992) found that people with schizophrenia from many developing societies had quicker and more complete recovery than did those from more industrialized societies. It seems plausible that this may stem in part from the cultural differences in the attributions and EE levels expressed from their family members and from the other emotional responses that follow.

However, an important consideration when reviewing the EE literature is the cultural norms of the countries in which a categorization of high or low EE is made. For example, Heresco-Levy and colleagues (1990) find that anger is more openly expressed in Israel and restraint of expression is seen as a weakness, and therefore criticism and hostility may be more commonly expressed among these populations in general. Similarly, emotional overinvolvement is common among Indian and Jewish cultures (Bhugra & McKenzie, 2003). Therefore, it is not surprising that the research finding a negative impact of high EE on schizophrenia outcomes is varied (Singh, Harley, & Suhail, 2013). Culture greatly influences an individual's experience of EE. Hence, among cultures in which certain EE attributes are norms, EE should be carefully operationalized. Researchers have recommended that EE be placed within a cultural context and norms be considered before generalizing the association to relapse in schizophrenia (Bhugra & McKenzie, 2003; Cheng, 2002). This is particularly important given that some studies assess EE across cultures but do not directly assess illness outcomes (Sadath, Kumr, & Karlsson, 2018).

## The Importance of Collectivism

Early research in this area (e.g., Lefley, 1990; Weisman, 1997) speculated that strong family values and a collectivistic orientation may underlie the lower rates of high EE among traditional cultures and the more benign course observed for schizophrenia patients from these societies. *Collectivism* refers to a social pattern in which members perceive themselves as part of a collective (e.g., family, co-workers, tribe, nation). With this perception comes a greater willingness to prioritize the goals of the group over the self, a sense of connectedness with other members, and motivation to abide by the norms and duties of the collective (Triandis, 1995/2018).

Previous work (Singelis, 1994; Sedikides, Gaertner, & Toguchi, 2003) suggests that, compared to a strong value placed on independence and uniqueness in mainstream American culture, many cultural groups emphasize interdependence and connectedness with others. The perception of being interconnected with another may lead to empathy for one's problems and, in turn, to more supportive reactions; positive associations between empathy and collectivistic beliefs have been found (Duan, Wei, & Wang, 2008; Heinke & Luis, 2009), and this connection appears to be stronger in more collectivistic groups like H/Ls (Segal et al., 2011). This may be particularly true for individuals sharing genetic ties. This empathetic response may also prove beneficial to the "giver." Enacting behavior consistent with one's orientation is related to positive self-belief (Sedikides et al., 2003).

In H/L cultures, as is true for many traditional cultural groups, the family is considered to be the single most important social unit for the individual (Cauce & Domenech-Rodríguez, 2002; Rodriguez, Mira, Paez, & Myers, 2007). This is true for other ethnic minority groups as well (Almeida, 2005; Barakat, 2004). It seems reasonable that individuals with strongly familistic (i.e., subordinating personal interests and prerogatives of an individual to the values and demands of the family) identities might be motivated to view the odd or disruptive behaviors of a loved one in a more benign way to preserve the solidarity of the family. In line with this, in a qualitative analysis of 24 relatively unacculturated H/L caregivers of a family member with schizophrenia in the United States, Weisman, Gomes, and Lopez (2003) found that nearly all participants expressed attributions that shifted blame away from their family member with mental illness. Believing that the relative with schizophrenia is unable to control disruptive behaviors may help justify and facilitate continued acceptance of the family members in the household.

Drawing from this and other research, it seems that strong family and religious values and a tendency to externalize blame may be two factors underlying the greater compassion and lower rates of criticism from Hispanic relatives (and perhaps other minority groups) toward their loved ones with schizophrenia. Strengthening these values and beliefs in treatment programs may help people with SSDs and their relatives to better cope with mental illness. Moreover, these benefits are likely to occur for minority and nonminority families alike.

## The Importance of Religion and Spirituality

Historically, clinicians have avoided utilizing religion/spirituality in treating individuals with schizophrenia due to concern about reinforcing religious delusions. However, not all individuals experience this symptom and many individuals with schizophrenia have normative religious/spiritual beliefs that are being underutilized as a tool to assist in managing symptoms and promoting adherence to medication (Grover, Davuluri, & Chakrabarti, 2014). Consequently, we should not overlook the abundance of research supporting the benefits of religion on mental health outcomes. For example, being religious has been found to be associated with better social and emotional functioning when dealing with difficult life events (Pargament, Koenig, Tarakeshwar, & Hahn, 2004). Moreover, Sanders and colleagues (2015) found that religiousness, spiritual maturity, and self-transcendence were significantly predictive of better mental health outcomes and positive functioning, which included decreased depression, anxiety, and obsessive-compulsive features. Furthermore, greater religiosity was predictive of greater self-esteem, identity integration, moral self-approval, and meaning in life. Moreover, research has found that perceived support from religious sources mediates the relationship between experienced racial microaggressions and general psychological well-being (Kim, 2017). These findings are all consistent with the present literature on spirituality and religiosity as associated with positive mental health status and greater psychosocial functioning.

One reason why CIT-S focuses on culture and aims to increase ethnic pride is because there is mounting evidence that doing so is associated with greater well-being, particularly among ethnic minorities. Several researchers have examined different acculturation approaches and their relationships to mental health. According to Berry (2005), acculturation refers to the dual process of cultural and psychological change that takes place as a result of contact between two or more cultural groups and their individual members. From years of research in this area (Berry, 2006; Sam & Berry, 2006), Berry has developed a framework that posits four discrete acculturation strategies for bicultural individuals.

- The first strategy, *integration*, refers to valuing and engaging with the host society while also maintaining a strong minority cultural identity.
- The second strategy, *assimilation*, refers to relinquishing the minority culture and primarily engaging in and valuing relationships and activities with only the host society.
- The third strategy, *separation*, refers to maintaining the minority culture but living with very little to no interaction with those from the host culture.
- The final approach, *marginalization*, refers to establishing a limited number of relationships with those in the host culture but also relinquishing many of the values and traditions from one's culture of origin.

Not surprisingly, in several studies on nonpsychiatric samples (Berry, 2005, 2006; Berry & Sabatier, 2010; Sam & Berry, 2006), integration was found to be the approach with the most positive psychological well-being followed by assimilation, separation, and, finally, marginalization as the least adaptive strategy.

Weisman de Mamani and colleagues (2017) examined Berry's model in a sample of 128 H/L and Black individuals with schizophrenia. In line with the model and Berry's earlier findings, the acculturation strategy predicted quality of life with the highest levels for those in the integrated category (i.e., those who maintained strong pride and ethnic identity associated with the minority culture but also valued and interacted with those of the host culture) and the lowest for those in the marginalized group, with those in the assimilated and separation groups falling in between. Other research also indicates that ethnic pride is associated with well-being. For example, Kiang, Yip, Gonzales-Backen, Witkow, and Fuligni (2006) examined protective effects of ethnic identity on the daily psychological well-being of 415 ninth graders of Mexican and Chinese backgrounds living in the United States. They found that adolescents who had greater regard for their ethnic group exhibited greater levels of happiness and lower levels of anxiety over a two-week period.

## Evidence Supporting CIT-S

CIT-S is a manualized psychotherapy approach that was informed by the research cited in Chapter 1 of this volume. The intervention draws heavily from established cognitive-behavioral approaches/techniques (Dickerson, 2004; for manual see Kingdon & Turkington, 2005) in that a main goal is to help clients carefully examine their thoughts, behaviors, and emotions and to better understand the connections between them. Clients are then helped to reshape maladaptive thoughts and modify behaviors to help them better manage mental illness and live their lives in a manner that aligns with and draws from their cultural beliefs and values. We have now published several papers that have evaluated different aspects of the intervention. Our overarching findings indicate strong empirical support for the efficacy of the intervention. For example,

- As expected, CIT-S proved more effective than a psychoeducation-only comparison condition in reducing psychiatric symptoms, with a medium effect size (Weisman, Weintraub, Gurak, & Maura, 2014).
- Also in line with expectations, Maura and Weisman de Mamani (2018) found that CIT-S was effective in reducing psychiatric symptoms in people with schizophrenia in a multifamily group version of the intervention, although the comparison condition for this study was a waitlist control rather than an active comparison condition.
- We further found that CIT-S outperformed a psychoeducation-only condition in reducing caregiver burden, with a large effect size (Weisman de Mamani & Suro, 2016).

■ Furthermore, as hypothesized, CIT-S has demonstrated superiority to a psychoeducation-only comparison condition in reducing depression, anxiety, and stress in both patients and caregivers (Brown & Weisman de Mamani, 2018). In this same study and in line with treatment goals, Brown and Weisman Mamani (2018) also found that CIT-S increased family cohesion and this change appeared to mediate the treatment effect on psychiatric symptoms.

Contrary to expectations, in another study (Gurak, Weisman de Mamani, & Ironson, 2017), we found that clients who were more religious dropped out of treatment earlier and more often than did less religious participants. This was surprising given that CIT-S directly targets religiosity during the third module of the intervention. However, results of a survival analysis indicated that nearly all participants who left the treatment prematurely did so before the religiosity segment began. In fact, no participants dropped out of treatment after completing the religiosity module. Thus, CIT-S may have been too compartmentalized and religious individuals may have perceived a disconnection between their beliefs and those of their mental health providers. Based on these findings we have modified CIT-S to better integrate religion throughout the intervention by opening and closing each session with a prayer and by incorporating religious techniques throughout the intervention. As a related project, we currently have a pilot study underway, funded by the John Templeton Foundation, to develop a group version of culturally informed therapy that will be available to people with a wide range of disorders (anxiety, depression, substance use). We are offering one arm of the intervention in a religious institution with the aim of improving retention of religious participants.

## Structure of CIT-S

The intervention was developed and tested by Amy Weisman de Mamani, the first author of this clinician guide, and her research team. To reiterate, CIT-S is not tied to any specific ethnic or cultural group and is instead uniquely tailored to the beliefs, values, and traditions of the participants being served. Throughout this book, we offer case examples and information that illustrate how the intervention can be tailored to people from different cultural backgrounds. The intervention includes the following five modules, each lasting three sessions, for 15 weekly sessions: (a) family collectivism, (b) psychoeducation, (c) spirituality, (d) communication training, and (e) problem-solving. The psychoeducation, communication training, and problem-solving modules were influenced heavily by prior therapies for schizophrenia and bipolar disorders (e.g., Falloon, Boyd, & McGill, 1984; Goldstein & Miklowitz, 1994). We will provide further rationale for these modules in Chapters, 4, 6, and 7. We have found 60 minutes per session to be optimal for most families, although for large families with multiple participating members or for more challenging cases, 75 minutes may be warranted. Figure 2.1 illustrates an overview of CIT-S.

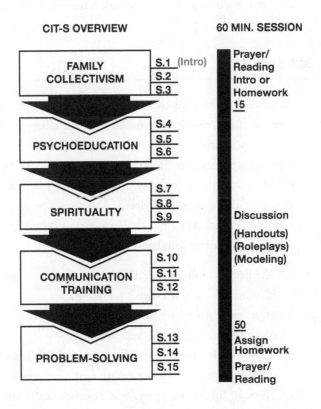

**Figure 2.1**

Overview of CIT-S.

The first session of collectivism is also an introduction to CIT-S as a whole. During the first treatment session, give participants a general orientation to treatment, including clinician goals and responsibilities as well as expectations of participants. Handout 2: *Culturally Informed Therapy for Schizophrenia* (see the appendix at the end of this clinician guide) should be given to participants so that they may follow along as you discuss the roles and expectations of the clinician and family members, treatment goals, and session format. This handout explains each of these areas in detail, and you can choose to read the points of the handout aloud and follow each with a brief explanation. To encourage a reciprocal dialogue between you and the participants and to avoid a situation in which you are doing all the talking, it is important to make several pauses to allow participants to ask questions or make comments. By modeling collectivistic behavior, you establish a precedent that encourages full participation from all members.

## Organization of Each Section

As noted earlier in this chapter, we recommend each session begin with a religious and/or spiritual component. For example, you can start the session by asking family members if any of them would like to offer a prayer or intention. If someone offers, then the rest of the group members can listen (or pray along). Other examples include asking group members to read a scripture or discuss a positive religious experience they had in the past week. Each session (beginning with Session 2) should be organized as follows:

- The first few minutes should be used to discuss, examine, and troubleshoot the previous week's homework.
- Next, present new session material and ask family members to discuss this with each other and with you.
- Third, family members should practice, through discussion or structured exercises, the implementation of these concepts.
- Through further role plays and exercises, assist family members to apply these concepts to their own family interactions.
- Finally, assign homework to increase generalization of the concepts to real-life situations.

During each phase of CIT-S, concepts should be introduced slowly to help reduce participants' anxiety and to increase generalization of both skills and ideas. Ideally, you should present CIT-S material in a conversational interactive manner, rather than didactically. Handouts are provided as guides to each session; you do not need to ask every question, and in many cases this material is addressed naturally during conversation. Take care to adjust terminology and the presentation of materials to the educational background of the family.

## Important Additional Considerations

As illustrated in the first two chapters, culture can influence the course of mental illness and family functioning. Furthermore, competently addressing culture in therapy can be an asset for clients suffering from SSDs and for their family members. In chapters 3 to 7, we will break down each CIT-S module and give detailed examples of how it can be applied to clients of diverse backgrounds.

Before describing the specific modules, we would like to underscore that every client and family is distinct. Thus, it is important for you to take the family's unique cultural background into account during all aspects of CIT-S. This includes examining their conceptions of mental illness and their understanding of symptoms (as noted in Chapter 4), and gauging how they interpret their religious (Chapter 5) and other cultural practices and beliefs. In CIT-S, it is not the clinician's role to teach clients about their culture. On the contrary, we view clients as the experts on their own culture and the clinician's role is to draw out and synthesize this information. In other words, CIT-S is designed to be client specific and addresses clients' unique views of their culture and the beliefs, values, and traditions that are important to them. This information is then used to help clients manage their illness in a way that is in line with their beliefs and values, as well as the behaviors and traditions that are important to them.

We believe it is helpful for clinicians to attempt to gain a broad understanding of the history, philosophies, and typical customs of the primary ethnic, racial, and other cultural groups that they see frequently in practice. However, it is also important to keep in mind that even within individuals from the same broad ethnic or religious groups, there is often a great deal of variability in how each person conceptualizes their own culture. Therefore, we encourage clinicians to rely heavily on their clients, who are undoubtedly experts on their own culture, and who are in the best position to enlighten the clinician. We hope that this understanding is comforting in that it would be difficult, if not impossible, to become thoroughly grounded in the *culture* of all of the different types of clients (e.g., ethnic, racial, sexual orientation/identity) that you are likely to encounter in your lifetime.

Finally, and in the same vein, it is important to highlight that nearly all clients have multiple intersecting identities. Thus, each client's cultural beliefs and values are likely to be complex and unique from that of other individuals with overlapping identities. For example, Adames, Chavez-Dueñas, Sharma, and La Roche (2018) note that the literature on H/L identity often focuses on ethnicity but neglects the role of race in the lives of individuals of H/L descent. Similarly, the same group of authors observed that the literature examining sexual orientation and gender diversity among H/L tends to focus more heavily on the role of sexual orientation and culture, without explicitly considering the role of ethnicity or race in the lives of the Lesbian, Gay, Bisexual, Transgender, and Queer (LGBTQ) community. Thus, in CIT-S (and in most other psychotherapy approaches), it is important to ask clients about their multiple intersecting identities and to guard against making perfunctory assumptions about clients. This often requires clinicians to reflect on their own cultural beliefs, expectations, or biases and to guard against unintentionally imposing these on clients.

# CHAPTER 3

# Module 1—Family Collectivism (Sessions 1–3)

## Handouts for This Module

Refer to Table 3.1 later in this chapter for suggestions on how to break the module into three sessions and which handout(s) to use for each session.

- Handout 1: Culturally Informed Therapy for Schizophrenia
- Handout 2: Family Dynamics

## Background Information for the Clinician

As stated earlier, the importance placed on individualism in the United States is not shared by many other cultures or by U.S. minority groups, which emphasize humility, anonymity, and a submission of the self to the welfare of one's group (both the family and the community). According to Aponte and Johnson (2000), the intense focus on the individual that is typical of mainstream U.S. therapies is alien to these world views. They caution that a lack of sensitivity to the discomfort induced in ethnic or cultural minorities by such factors can lead to ineffective treatment and early termination.

As noted in Chapter 1 of this volume, the strength of the family, in particular, has often been regarded as especially important for individuals from traditional cultures. Asian Americans, for example, tend to be highly group-oriented. They place a strong emphasis on family connection and view it as the major source of identity and the foundation for the development and understanding of one's ethnic background (Moua & Lamborn, 2010). The family model is an extended one including immediate family and relatives, and loyalty to the family is expected (Nguyen, Wong, & Juang, 2015). Thus, both family therapy and an emphasis on bolstering collectivism are especially well-suited to this group.

For Hispanic, Latino/a or Latinx (H/L) individuals, the family also holds an extremely important and valuable role and is often a focal point in their lives (Acosta, 1982; Barrio, Hernandez, & Barragan, 2011; Turcios-Cotto & Milan, 2013). The Latinos in America (2000) study suggests that the findings are generalizable to H/Ls of all backgrounds. Thus, while there are certainly differences among H/Ls of different countries of origin, the importance of the family seems to be a commonality among them. For clinicians aiming to establish credibility and trust when working with H/Ls and other minority groups, it is important to respect and incorporate the members of the extended family and to understand significant aspects of family relations. One such aspect is that of hierarchical patterns based on age and gender and of the individual's sense of their own boundaries as fluid and interconnected with those of their kin.

There is some evidence that family-oriented, interdependent approaches may be particularly effective with minority clients. Perhaps the best example comes from research by Szapocznik and associates (e.g., Szapocznik & Kurtines, 1993), primarily with Cuban American families. Szapocznik and colleagues have developed specific techniques to treat a variety of problems and disorders (e.g., adolescent drug abuse, depression in the elderly, HIV-infected gay Hispanic males) using a systems approach that incorporates Cuban values. In a landmark paper, Szapocznik and Kurtines (1993) describe viewing clients' problems within a contextualist paradigm. *Contextualism* refers to the view that behavior cannot be understood outside of the context in which it occurs. Contextualism is concerned with the interaction between the organism and the environment. In sum, research by Organista and Muñoz (1996), Szapocznik et al. (1993), and others (Gutiérrez-Maldonado & Caqueo-Urízar, 2007; Barrio & Yamada, 2010) indicates that behaviorally oriented, psychoeducational programs that fortify culturally sanctioned coping mechanisms such as spirituality, collectivism, and family unity may improve the functioning of H/L individuals dealing with mental illness in the family.

Family collectivism is the first module of CIT-S and lasts three sessions. You may wish to refer to Chapter 2 of this volume to give an appropriate introduction and explanation for CIT-S as a whole during the first session. This discussion should be guided using Handout 1: Culturally Informed Therapy for Schizophrenia.

---

*Clinician Note*

*All handouts can be found in the appendix at the end of this therapist guide. You may photocopy the handouts for your clients, or you may download these items from the Treatments That Work Web site at www.oxfordclinincalpsych.com/CITS.*

---

## Introducing Module 1: Family Collectivism

The first phase of treatment, family collectivism, is aimed at fortifying a strong sense of family unity and helping members to view themselves as a team working toward a mutual goal. In the first session, commend each family member for coming to treatment. Frame this reinforcement as indicating a real commitment to the person with a schizophrenia spectrum disorder (SSD) and to the family. Ask participants what they hope to gain from the treatment and point out commonalities. For instance, most family members and those with an SSD will likely report that they hope to see improvement in the functioning of the family member with a mental illness. Also, ask family members to describe their perceptions of their roles in the family. That is, ask them to discuss their beliefs about how they contribute to the family, both in terms of enhancing family well-being and possibly contributing to family problems. These and several other topics for discussion can be found in Handout 2: Family Dynamics, which should be distributed to participants following the introduction to CIT-S, which is described in Chapter 2 of this volume.

Following Szapocznik and Kurtines (1993), participants should be encouraged to view themselves as a system of interdependent and interrelated individuals whose behaviors necessarily affect other family members. Differences in generational and gender roles should be discussed. In session or for homework, ask participants to prepare narratives (either written or audiotaped) that they can share in treatment. These narratives should describe how each member thinks that they might contribute differently to improve family functioning. In addition, encourage them to point out specific behaviors in other members that they appreciate and think enhance family well-being, as well as behaviors that they would like to see increased or modified to better benefit the family as a whole. Utilize these narratives in the early sessions primarily to help families get a clearer picture of how each member contributes and influences the family system and to generate ideas about potentially improving family functioning.

These narratives sometimes generate feelings of anger as participants identify problem behaviors in other family members. Be sure to provide families with a transcultural perspective that emphasizes commonalities between members and de-emphasizes differences. Make an effort to deflect the blame for family problems away from any one individual (e.g., the person with an SSD). However, do not formally instruct families to implement any changes to their behavior based on these narratives until the fourth (communication training) and fifth (problem-solving) phases of treatment, when the ideas generated from the narratives are revisited. For example, some families may have conflict surrounding gender identity, sexual orientation, or relationship orientation (monogamous, nonmonogamous), such as a parent refusing to use the pronoun or new gender affirming name that a trans client has adopted for themselves. This is an opportunity for you to affirm the pronouns and/or preferred terms of the individual, while connecting familial concerns to surrounding culture. Acknowledging conflicting beliefs (e.g., belief that actions are sinful versus belief that actions are benign) and then focusing and spending more time on shared values (e.g., unconditional love, family loyalty, desire for closeness) can assist families in shifting their perspective such that they are focused on shared goals.

In this module, you should set a ground rule early on that even when family members disagree with one another, they should listen attentively to everyone's point of view and respect beliefs and values that may differ from one's own. This will help maintain a cohesive family environment and will be especially helpful in later modules, where clients often hold important differences of view on religious beliefs, values, and other issues that arise in the communication training and problem-solving modules. It is helpful in later sessions to refer to this ground rule should tensions escalate among family members.

Finally, throughout this module (and CIT-S as a whole), participants are encouraged to engage in traditions from their cultural backgrounds as a family to increase ethnic pride and to bolster their sense of connection with one another and with other members of their ethnic, racial, or other cultural community. For example, if clients like food from their background, you might encourage them to cook an ethnic meal together. If they enjoy the music from their culture, you might suggest they attend a concert or sing and dance to the music together. If there is a particular game (e.g., mahjong, chess) or sport (e.g., rugby) that they like and that is connected to their cultural heritage, you could suggest that they set aside a regular time to play as a family. Not only is this useful in building a sense of team spirit and family cohesion, it can also bolster ethnic pride, which we noted in Chapter 2 of this volume as being associated with better quality of life (Weisman et al., 2017) and better well-being (Berry, 2005, 2006; Berry & Sabatier, 2010; Kiang et al., 2006; Sam & Berry, 2006).

## Additional Considerations and Conclusions

Because caring for a relative with schizophrenia can be burdensome, many families will express interest when offered the chance to participate in a treatment program that purports to help the person with an SSD as well as the rest of the family. However, some families might be hesitant to try yet another intervention and may be skeptical that a psychotherapeutic treatment can actually help with a disorder that, as they have likely been told, is mainly biological. Other families may be cautious because they feel a stigma attached to having a family member with a mental illness, and being in therapy only reminds them of that stigma. Therefore, one goal during the first few sessions is to engage the interest of the family and to alleviate any of their initial concerns. Highlighting in CIT-S that we value the family, that we will work with them to combat the stigma, and that this treatment has the empirical backing to give us the confidence that we can help them manage the symptoms and improve the quality of their lives may help in this regard.

## Dividing Module 1 Into Three Sessions

Table 3.1 is a guideline for how the three sessions can be divided in Module 1. As with all modules, some families will master certain tasks more easily than others. Similarly, some families will benefit from spending more time on one topic than another, or avoiding some topics altogether. Thus, we want to underscore that this is only an example of a session-by-session breakdown. We encourage you to adapt session content and flow based on clients' needs. It is important to note that each of the three sessions should begin with a prayer, followed by homework review, and end with a homework assignment from either the following list or another appropriate alternative.

**Table 3.1 Sample Guidelines for Breaking Module 1 Into Three Sessions**

| Module 1 | | | |
|---|---|---|---|
| | **Session 1** | **Session 2** | **Session 3** |
| **Handouts** | 1: Culturally Informed Therapy for Schizophrenia | 2. Family Dynamics | 2. Family Dynamics |
| **Content** | – Introductions<br>– Overview of CIT-S<br>– Address client reservations about treatment<br>– Emphasize family commonalities and the goal of enhancing family cohesion and team spirit | – Discuss topics on Handout 2 with the aim of better understanding functional and dysfunctional family patterns, traditions, etc. | – Discuss client views of their ideal family<br>– Set goals and discuss strategies that can be implemented in future modules to achieve these goals |

## Suggested Family Collectivism Homework Assignments

After having introduced the Family Collectivism Module and the general framework of this approach, for homework:

- Ask the family to brainstorm together the commonalities they share and what they appreciate about each member. Encourage family members to avoid discussing flaws in others or what they may be lacking until after they have focused on aspects that they do appreciate.
- Ask the family to write descriptions of how they see the family structure and the roles of each member of the family. Members should be told to do this slowly throughout the week, as they notice family actions and needs, not in one day solely off memory or opinion. Some roles that may be discussed in preparation for the homework are the sick role, the protector, the mediator, the reliable person, the fixer, and the head of the family. Ask members to consider their cultural values and beliefs and whether certain roles are dictated by their culture.
- Have clients block out a time to sit together as a family to discuss how each member feels about their roles, how they may change if they feel unsatisfied in their role/s, and how they may modify their roles and behaviors to help improve overall family functioning.
- Encourage families to engage in traditions from their cultural backgrounds (e.g., salsa dancing, making a Chinese hot pot, listening to jazz, or hip hop) as a family to increase ethnic pride and their sense of connection with one another and with their ethnic community outside of the home. To avoid stereotyping, never suggest specific activities that they may enjoy. Instead, ask the members questions about what activities are common in their culture to help them identify these on their own and decide which ones they might enjoy doing together.

## Family Collectivism: Case Illustration

Jia, her husband Hwan, and their daughter Jin, originally from South Korea, attended CIT-S after seeing an advertisement on the subway. The family moved to the United States seven years ago, when Hwan's work had transferred him to a position within their New York branch. At that time, Jin was 19. Following the cross-country move, Jin began to develop symptoms of schizophrenia including paranoia, social withdrawal, and auditory hallucinations. Her parents reported that at first they took these symptoms to be her response to such a big life change. They considered that Jin might be depressed, but after her symptoms worsened and she began to accuse her mother of spying on her at school and putting sedatives in her food, Jia and Hwan realized Jin was experiencing something more severe. They pulled her out of school, as she was also struggling to attend classes due to her paranoia, and tried to help her at home as much as they could. However, after three years of trying to cope with the disorder within the family, Jin's paranoia escalated, and Jia and Hwan felt they could no longer help their daughter on their own. Eventually, they took Jin to the hospital after they found her speaking to herself saying she "didn't want to do it" as she held a handful of pills in her palm. At the hospital, she was diagnosed with schizophrenia and prescribed antipsychotic medication. With medication, there was a drastic reduction in her symptoms. However, she continued to struggle with low level symptoms and remained greatly dependent on her parents for social, financial, and emotional support.

On his way to work one day, Hwan saw an advertisement for CIT-S. He was intrigued by the description of "a religiously based, culturally informed, cognitive behavioral intervention for schizophrenia," as Jin's symptoms had not fully receded and the family strongly identify as Christian. Jia and Hwan have prayed for Jin to get better and believe that God has helped them through the most difficult times. Jin and her family were hoping that integration of their spiritual understanding and psychological coping techniques in CIT-S would be the help they needed.

The Family Collectivism Module was initiated by a discussion of the benefits that community and social contact have on mental health, with the clinician highlighting the social nature of humans, the need to communicate and share time with others, the comfort of feeling supported by various people, and the benefits of shared activities. The family resonated with this. All three agreed that community and family are of great importance to them and are the bedrocks of Korean culture. Jin explained that, in Korean culture, family is an integral part of life, and family members are taught that they should help one another and treat each other with mutual respect.

The family reported being excited to engage in a treatment that specifically targeted these values.

Upon arriving to the second session, Jia gave an elegantly wrapped box, which contained a traditional Korean silk dress, to the clinician. Although the clinician normally did not accept expensive gifts from clients, gift-giving is a common social practice within Korean culture and would be expected in many contexts similar to this. Moreover, to reject the gift in this situation could be viewed as disrespectful and could work against the collective and cohesive climate that the clinician was trying to create. Therefore, she graciously accepted the gift and welcomed the family to the session. This gesture appeared to increase her bond with the family.

During the Family Collectivism Module, the clinician worked from questions in the handouts. For example, the family members discussed what community and family meant to each family member and what roles and structures each person played in their family. All three members agreed that there was a clear hierarchy in their family, with Hwan on top as the breadwinner, followed by Jia who maintains the household, and lastly, Jin, as the daughter.

Jia discussed how important family is to her and how she sees her role as the glue that holds her family together. She mentioned that she strives to be a good mother and a good wife, always preparing food, keeping the home clean, and being present for her family when needed. Jin reported feeling that her role was that of family "failure" because she believed that a good daughter is someone who is able to support her family, especially as they age, yet she felt certain that she would always be the family member who needed the most help. Moreover, Jin reported being fearful that she would never marry or have children and would therefore let her family down even further. The clinician asked Jin why she thought that not being married was such a let-down to her family. Jin described that marrying is what a respectful daughter should do in Korea. She mentioned that one of the best contributions a daughter can make is to bring a successful son-in-law into the family. Jin reported being fearful that, because of her illness, she would remain unmarried and a burden on her parents. Jin's parents responded with surprise. Jia and Hwan explained that while they wanted Jin to be happy, to someday marry, and to have children, they also viewed having their only child live at home with them as a blessing. They added that they would actually miss her terribly when she eventually married and moved out.

In addition to the perceived failure of remaining unmarried, Jin reported feeling like a failure because of her illness. She expressed concern that she brought too much trouble to the family and felt guilty for disrespecting her parents when she was highly symptomatic and paranoid. She began to describe what she felt she had done but struggled to find the words in English. She mentioned that her mother and father's *Kibun* (Korean term with no literal translation but thought to be related to the emotions of pride and dignity; Robinson & Fisher, 1992) had been damaged. She said there was a loss of harmony and balance in the family after these incidents. Moreover, she felt she did not contribute at all to her family and felt great shame because of it. Hwan, on the other hand, thought he had failed Jin as a father and blamed himself for her illness because he saw it as partly due to the stress he inflicted by his work relocation.

The clinician asked each member to share their perception of the other members' roles and their strengths. The family was receptive and each relayed how important each of the other members is to them. Jia spoke of how much she cherished her father and how his strength helped her through hard times. Hwan stated that Jin was not Jin when she was very symptomatic, but rather her actions were guided by her illness. He expressed to Jin that he valued her as a daughter and that although he also worried about her future, he was confident that they would figure it out together. For homework, the family was assigned the task of closely monitoring and assessing the daily contributions that each member made to the family.

In the next session, the clinician asked if one member would like to open the session with a prayer. Jia volunteered and read the prayer: "Help us be thankful for one another. Help our family to be thankful for each member and to pray for one another continually. Our gratitude for each other will bind us as a family and our prayers for each other will unify us in gratitude and love." Thereafter, the clinician asked about last week's homework regarding individual family members' contributions to the family. Hwan volunteered to go first and stated that his contributions included financial stability for the family, love for his wife and daughter, and instrumental support. He noted that in the past week he helped fix his wife's jewelry drawer that was stuck after he noticed her repeated frustration trying to open it. He reported that he had not thought much about fixing it (he took fixing the drawer for granted) until he saw Jia light up with relief after she was finally able to open it. Hwan mentioned that he provides small moments like those for his family.

Jin noted that this assignment made her even more aware of her dependence on her parents during the week. She was unable to find any contributions that she felt she had made to her family. She reported being distraught by the realization of just how much her parents aid her in daily life and how little she gives back.

To attempt to lift Jin's distress, the clinician asked Hwan and Jia if they had noticed any contributions made by Jin in the past week. Hwan mentioned that Jin always helps Jia prepare dinner. Jin discredited that by saying this is an expectation of a daughter, not a contribution. The clinician then asked Jin to describe some ideal contributions that she would like to make to her family. After a moment, Jin stated that she would like to have a husband and not be a burden on her family. The clinician asked Jin to brainstorm other possibilities for contributing on a daily basis. Jin mentioned that she should be respectful, kind, and grateful toward her parents. The clinician asked Jia and Hwan if they felt similarly. Both parents said they feel that Jin is very grateful and respectful toward them. Hwan further stated that the illness is a burden upon Jin and their entire family but made the important distinction that Jin herself is not a burden. The clinician asked Jia what she thought Jin was capable of doing that could help her contribute more to the family. Jia responded that Jin should be going to church socials and to events at the Korean American Club to find a good husband. The clinician then asked if there is anything else she could think of that Jin could be doing on a daily basis. Jia reported that Jin actually helps a lot with the daily cooking and cleaning and felt that there really isn't much more that she (or any other daughter) could be doing. She added that Jin often reminds her of important things that need to get done at home, as her own memory has started to slip here and there. Jia stated that, overall, she mainly feels concerned about Jin's future marriage prospects, but otherwise feels content with Jin and their relationship.

The clinician took this opportunity to highlight the fact that all members appear to value the family unit and each other. Furthermore, all members appear to be contributing meaningfully to family functioning and recognize these contributions in each other, yet each family member appears to be their own harshest critic. The clinician reiterated that all three members highlighted strengths and contributions of all other members. Therefore, an important focus moving forward would be to build on the strengths that each member already has and to work together toward shared goals, such as extending their family by helping Jin to find a life partner. The clinician mentioned that keeping Jin's symptoms in check would be very important in achieving this goal and that they would discuss symptom management much more extensively in the following module (psychoeducation).

# CHAPTER 4

# Module 2— Psychoeducation (Sessions 4–6)

## Handouts for This Module

Refer to Table 4.1 later in this chapter for suggestions on how to break the module into three sessions and which handout(s) to use for each session.

- Handout 3: Schizophrenia in the Context of Culture
- Handout 4: Symptoms of Schizophrenia
- Handout 5: Other Common Mental Health Concerns
- Handout 6: How Does Schizophrenia Develop?
- Handout 7: Course of Schizophrenia
- Handout 8: What Can the Family Do to Assist?

## Background Information for the Clinician

White and Marsella (1982) were pioneers in exporting the notion that illness experience is an *interpretive* enterprise, which is constructed in social situations according to the premises of cultural "theories" about illness and social behavior more generally. This can easily be applied to mental illness in that research has long suggested that there is wide variation across countries and cultures in determining what mental illness is and in the application of giving a mental illness diagnosis. Moreover, research suggests that cultural perceptions around mental illness along with other factors associated with cultural norms (e.g., mental illness stigma), determine clients' and clinician's views on effective routes to treatment (Baskin, 1984; Weisman de Mamani et al., 2020). Thus, presenting mental illness information in culturally sensitive ways that incorporate clients' own beliefs and values around schizophrenia spectrum disorders (SSDs) is essential to ensuring their willingness to engage in treatment and their receptiveness to the specific information and techniques used in psychotherapy. In this section, we discuss methods of presenting didactic information about SSDs in a manner that is culturally competent and likely to be appealing to clients from diverse ethnic and cultural backgrounds.

The primary objective of culturally informed therapy for schizophrenia (CIT-S), and psychoeducation in particular, is to impart information and techniques that will help improve the mental health and functioning of people with SSDs and their family members. Based on past psychoeducational programs (e.g., Falloon, Boyd, & McGill, 1984; Goldstein & Miklowitz, 1994), we believe that one crucial factor involved in achieving this goal is to educate clients about the nature of schizophrenia, the known triggers, and protective factors associated with relapse prevention and functioning. It is important to teach clients about their symptoms and their illness using up-to-date terminology. This will allow them to communicate more effectively with their mental and medical health providers and will also make them more informed consumers of mental illness websites and other educational material that can help them to better manage the illness.

The psychoeducational information in this section was heavily influenced by earlier family treatments for schizophrenia (Falloon et al., 1984) and bipolar disorder (Goldstein & Miklowitz, 1997). Material was updated and modified, especially with the aim of making it more relevant to ethnic, religious, and other cultural minorities. In line with the other modules of CIT-S, it is necessary to put this information in a language that makes sense to our clients and that fits within their own framework and understanding of mental illness. Although psychoeducation may appear to lend itself to a primarily didactic delivery of information, collaboration between clinician and clients is necessary to understand and address each member's cultural conceptualizations of schizophrenia and the associated symptoms and concerns that they may have regarding mainstream views of the illness and its treatment.

The duration of the psychoeducation phase is three sessions, and this module begins after the third session or upon completion of the Family Collectivism Module.

---

*Clinician Note*

*All handouts can be found in the appendix at the end of this therapist guide. You may photocopy the handouts for your clients, or you may download these items from the Treatments That Work Web site at www. oxfordclinincalpsych.com/CITS*

---

## Introducing Module 2: Psychoeducation

Offer a rationale for psychoeducation, as some families may not see the direct benefits of education and/or may express that they already know all about the illness. Explain to the family, "I am interested in learning about your views of the illness and treatment as well as presenting you with what research has taught us about the illness and what works well in terms of managing it." To begin this module, present Handout 3: Schizophrenia in the Context of Culture. Each family member should be asked how they view schizophrenia (or whatever SSD they have; e.g., schizoaffective disorder) and how their family and, more generally, their culture perceives the illness. Ask clients to reflect on whether or what aspects of the disorder are stigmatized in their culture and how this plays out (e.g., ask the family member with an SSD whether they have had any direct stigmatizing experiences related to their illness). Discuss family members' perceptions of the cause of the illness and effective routes for treatment, including their thoughts about taking psychotropic medication. When clients present alternative views of mental illness and effective treatment, you should attempt to maintain a welcoming and nonjudgmental stance toward the family and their views. This can be done in many ways. For example, a client might come from a culture where spiritual healers and special ceremonies are commonly used to treat mental illness. In this case, you might say something to the effect of "In my experience, spiritual practices and important cultural rituals can be very soothing to clients and can help them connect more strongly to one another and, as a result, can help better manage the illness." However, you can further point out that "despite these practices, your family is still experiencing struggles, or you would not have likely sought out this treatment." You could then reassure the family that "most people dealing with serious mental illness (even those coping well) benefit from professional help." You should then underscore that the techniques used in CIT-S are likely to complement practices that the family is already using.

In some cases, however, you will have to confront clients regarding cultural practices that are known to be detrimental (e.g., using hallucinogen drugs or other illicit substances). In these instances, explain the research, offer a rationale for why the practice is detrimental, and help the client or family substitute a more adaptive cultural practice to take its place. Examples of this are provided later in this chapter.

## Symptoms of Schizophrenia

Before beginning a discussion of the symptoms of schizophrenia, it can be helpful to say something to the effect of, "I know you've all been through a tough time, and the purpose of focusing on this material is to put your own experiences into a context that will make sense."

At this point, distribute Handout 4: Symptoms of Schizophrenia and explain the difference between "positive symptoms" and "negative symptoms" as well as review the definitions of each symptom. You should take care not to simply explain the symptoms mechanically. Instead, use this handout (and all handouts in CIT-S) to stimulate family-wide discussion. Encourage participants to not only discuss whether they have observed a specific symptom but also to discuss what that symptom symbolized for them. For example, in some cultures positive symptoms may be assumed to reflect possession by spirits or other mischievous creatures. As this belief can induce fear, sharing with clients the literature that strongly implicates the connection between faulty biochemistry and these symptoms cross-culturally can be helpful in this regard.

There are several reasons why participants should become very familiar with the symptoms of the disorder:

1. Having this information will make clients better able to identify the prodromal symptoms of new episodes, which will allow for more aggressive intervention.
2. Learning that the family member with mental illness has had many symptoms consistent with the diagnostic criteria for an SSD helps participants accept that the person suffers from a legitimate illness.
3. Understanding that the person has a legitimate illness helps family members to reframe previous faulty attributions that the symptomatic behaviors are due to "laziness," a desire to "get attention," or other potential misattributions.
4. Knowing the lingo will help family members communicate better with their health providers and will help them make better use of available published and Web-based resources.
5. Finally, learning that one is not alone, that their symptoms and disorder are common enough that they have a name, and that there are prescribed treatments to mitigate the symptoms and the disorder as a whole are often extremely reassuring to people with SSDs.

In the Psychoeducation Module, we also discuss associated symptoms that are common in people with schizophrenia but not necessarily hallmarks of the disorder, such as impaired memory and cognition and deficits in social cognition. You may suggest the use of mnemonic devices, list writing, and other techniques as a way to minimize the effect of poor memory or cognitive limitations on functioning. In this module, it is also important to note that symptoms of anxiety, depression, and stress are also common among people with SSDs and among their caregivers, and you can facilitate a discussion of these symptoms using Handout 5: Other Common Mental Health Concerns. We also encourage you to remind family members that prior research has indicated that the techniques used in CIT-S are not only effective in reducing schizophrenia symptoms but also in improving other aspects of mental health (lowering depression, anxiety, and stress) and in decreasing caregiver burden (Brown & Weisman de Mamani 2018; Weisman et al., 2014; Weisman de Mamani & Suro, 2016). Finally, we encourage you to draw from many established cognitive behavioral practices such as thinking traps, cognitive restructuring, and other cognitive-behavioral therapy

(CBT) methods (Sokol & Fox, 2019; Kingdon & Turkington, 2005) to address symptoms and potential maladaptive thoughts around having symptoms or having an SSD. As CBT is not unique to CIT-S, we highly suggest that you consider also using a manual for CBT in conjunction with this clinician guide for the application of these practices. For example, in this same Treatments That Work series, CBT manuals include *Mastery of Your Anxiety and Worry (MAW)* by Zinbarg, Craske, and Barlow (2006); *Overcoming Depression: A Cognitive Therapy Approach* by Gilson and Freeman (2009); and *Overcoming Your Alcohol or Drug Problem: Effective Recovery Strategies* by Daley and Marlatt (2006).

## How Do People Get Symptoms of Schizophrenia?

Once the participants have been acquainted with the symptoms of schizophrenia, you can begin to explain the reasons why the disorder occurs using Handout 6: How Does Schizophrenia Develop? This discussion may serve to reduce any guilt the family members may possess for having caused the disorder. As noted earlier, understanding the literature can also serve to address potential faulty attributions about symptoms (spirit possession) and therefore make such symptoms appear less frightening and mystical. Here, you will have another opportunity to explore the causal attributions for SSDs in the family's culture of origin and among members of their current home, work, and other environments in which they frequently find themselves.

Keep the following guidelines in mind when delivering etiological information to the family:

- Take a nonblaming, accepting stance.
- Talk about the multiple etiological pathways, including genetic, biological, and psychosocial factors.
- Do not accept the argument that any one factor (e.g., single person, event, or experience) caused the disorder.
- Emphasize the roles of protective as well as risk factors.
- Do not assume that genetic or biological explanations will always produce less guilt in family members than psychological ones, especially for a family member with a history of SSDs on their side of the family. Using a medical model analogy can be helpful here.

You can begin the discussion of etiological factors by saying: "Schizophrenia is caused by many factors that all interact with each other. No one person, event, or experience makes the disorder occur." You should explain that, as seen in Handout 6, stress interacts with a person's genetic and biological vulnerabilities or predispositions. That is, predispositions interact with how a person lives their life to determine whether or not the illness will manifest.

## Schizophrenia Across the Lifespan

The member with SSD and their family may wonder what this diagnosis means for them long term. Using Handout 7: Course of Schizophrenia, you should acknowledge that there are many courses of schizophrenia, and one individual may not look like the rest. You should also acknowledge each illness' trajectory and help families uncover concerns they may have about future psychotic episodes, illness severity, and other related topics. This is often a good time to identify signs and symptoms of relapse. While certain aspects of the family's situation may not be within their control (e.g., having the illness, being susceptible to psychotic episodes), stress that families can make decisions, nonetheless, that will improve their outcomes and the course of the illness.

## Family Involvement in Illness Management

To transition to the next handout, emphasize that no one factor (e.g., single person, event, or experience) is solely responsible for why someone becomes ill; however, there are things that the family can do to help the person cope with their mental illness. This discussion can be enhanced by providing Handout 8: What Can the Family Do to Assist? You may begin by encouraging family members to support the recommended treatment regimen (i.e., medication) for their relative and explain the role of medications in improving symptoms and preventing (and/or prolonging the time to) relapse. Many cultures discourage the use of psychotropic medication, so it is important to discuss each family member's perspective on how taking psychotropic medication is viewed in their culture. If there is hesitancy, it will be important to review the cross-cultural literature, which strongly shows that for the majority of people with SSDs around the world, the benefits of taking medication appear to greatly outweigh the costs (Ascher-Svanum et al., 2006; Leucht et al., 2009). It is also useful to obtain feedback from the person with the SSD as to what the family members can do to help their adherence to treatment.

Throughout the Psychoeducation Module, attributions and attitudes (i.e., expressed emotion) known to be associated with a poor course of illness are also directly targeted. Families are taught to develop balanced, realistic attributions regarding the amount of control people with SSDs have over the illness and its associated symptoms. Locus of control attributions are often deeply influenced by culture. Thus, exploring clients' controllability attributions about the illness and specific symptoms may be productive for opening the conversations around how many behaviors that may appear purposeful or characterological may, in fact, be core symptoms of mental illness. This may be especially helpful with respect to negative symptoms (e.g., poor hygiene), as research indicates that these types of symptoms were found to be criticized more often by family members than positive symptoms (Weisman, Nuechterlein, Goldstein, & Snyder, 1998). The authors contend that family members may be less tolerant of behavioral deficits, because they are more likely to be perceived as intentional, whereas the behavioral excesses are much more easily recognized as core symptoms of mental illness.

To begin this discussion, you may say something like:

> If you remember, using handouts 6-8, we discussed that people with the disorder do best when stress is kept to a minimum. This includes family stress. For example, when relatives are overly critical toward the individual with schizophrenia, or do not allow them enough independence, this creates stress for that person. Research shows that low-stress family environments for people with schizophrenia allow them to do much better over time, so a low-stress home can be a protective factor.

While we emphasize that families do not "cause" schizophrenia, family members can help after the onset with the implementation of protective factors. You will be teaching them that they can and should work together to overcome the illness. Participants learn about the detrimental effects of negatively charged home environments on both the individual with the SSD and their relatives. Furthermore, during the psychoeducation sessions you will also be addressing prosocial attitudes and behaviors, which are found to serve as protective factors against relapse. Specifically, clients learn how family unity and warmth may enhance functioning. Direct the family members to reflect on any attributions and attitudes (e.g., criticism, hostility) that may need reframing to maintain a warm and cohesive environment. To this aim, in this module and throughout CIT-S, encourage families to identify soothing activities that they can engage in together.

## Substance Abuse

We also place emphasis on educating participants about data strongly linking substance abuse, including alcohol and illicit substances (e.g., amphetamines) to schizophrenia relapse and poorer course of illness. This issue lends itself well to the discussion of culture and traditions in that many substance use problems are initiated and sustained by social and cultural rituals. For example, we have had more than one client explain that their consumption of wine (or in some cases other habits such as whiskey, cigars, cannabis, and cigarettes) began because of cultural rituals where libations and other substances were an important part of bonding customs around dinner and other celebrations. Many clients have described feeling that not partaking is a violation of their cultural traditions, and they worry that not engaging would be viewed as disrespectful or inconsiderate. This is a great opportunity to help clients tease apart the core experiences that they value (which in most cultures is connecting deeply with family and friends and being a productive member of their family and community) versus what may be the more superficial or distal ones (e.g., utilizing specific substances). Substance abuse often lends itself to the conversation that when people are using substances in excess, they are almost always less capable of managing their mental illness and other important aspects of their lives, such as the quality of their relationships. Thus, while engaging in substance abuse behaviors may be rewarding in the short run, it is generally at odds with participants' most pressing values and goals.

In CIT-S, for clients who are struggling with addictions (which is roughly half in schizophrenia; Swartz et al., 2006), we spend a lot of time helping them to establish alternative soothing (or exciting) rituals that may be more healthful substitutes. For example, a couple who had a weekend "healing" ritual of drinking tea made of peyote buttons while listening to ethnic drumming could instead be encouraged to maintain the ritual, but switch to a non-psychoactive herbal tea and perhaps enhance the service by adding incense or other agents to make it feel more ceremonial. For some clients, helping them establish new traditions altogether is effective as these may have fewer substance use memories associated with them and may therefore be less likely to trigger a relapse. One of the distinct benefits of family therapy is that members can help one another maintain substance-free behaviors by changing the home environment and helping one another establish newer, more adaptive pastimes.

## Additional Considerations and Conclusions

Upon completion of the Psychoeducation Module, participants should have a better, more comprehensive understanding of schizophrenia, including its signs and symptoms, how to recognize when these are recurring, what causes these symptoms to occur, and how the family can help temper symptoms. As a result, clients' anxieties and fears should be alleviated. Furthermore, the introduction of things family members can do to aid the person with an SSD will allow for the setting of goals in the later Communication Training and Problem-Solving Modules of the treatment.

## Dividing Module 2 into Three Sessions

Table 4.1 is a guideline for how the three sessions can be divided in Module 2. As with all modules, some families will master certain tasks more easily than others. Similarly, some families will benefit from spending more time on one topic than another or avoiding some topics altogether. For example, substance abuse might be a very salient topic for some families whereas for others who don't use at all, it may be

**Table 4.1 Sample Guidelines for Breaking Module 2 Into Three Sessions**

## Module 2

| | Session 1 | Session 2 | Session 3 |
|---|---|---|---|
| **Handouts** | 3: Schizophrenia in the Context of Culture | 6: How Does Schizophrenia Develop? | 8: What Can the Family Do to Assist? |
| | 4: Symptoms of Schizophrenia | 7: Course of Schizophrenia | 5: Other Common Mental Health Concerns |
| **Content** | • Discuss the family's conceptualizations of schizophrenia and their views on the causes and most effective routes for treatment | • Discuss genetic and biological causes of schizophrenia | • Discuss how the family can help their loved one with an SSD remain in remission by contributing to a low stress home environment |
| | • Review the symptoms of schizophrenia | • Review how biological factors interact with environmental factors to impact the course of the illness. | • Review symptoms of common comorbid disorders (depression, anxiety) and introduce thought monitoring and other CBT techniques to help family members cope with any symptoms they may be experiencing. |

*Notes:* CBT = cognitive-behavioral therapy; SSDs = schizophrenia spectrum disorders.

irrelevant. Thus, we want to underscore that this is only an example of a session-by-session breakdown. We encourage you to adapt session content and flow based on clients' needs. It is important to note that each of the three sessions should begin with a prayer, followed by homework review, and end with a homework assignment from either the following list or another appropriate alternative.

## Suggested Psychoeducation Homework Assignments

After having introduced the psychoeducation module and the biopsychosocial framework for understanding schizophrenia, for homework:

- Ask each family member to generate questions they have about the biological, psychological, or social underpinnings of schizophrenia. If family members believe there are other potential factors better explained by their culture (e.g., Santeria), facilitate their inquiries by endorsing a supportive and open environment.
- Ask family members to consider how cultural ideologies (e.g., *machismo,* independence) affect their current lives, particularly the way their loved one with schizophrenia operates as a member of that culture. For example, as a person with schizophrenia, does their gender or sexual orientation worsen, ameliorate, or have no effect on other aspects of life?
- Have clients write about what it means to be someone with serious mental illness in their culture. Ask them to think about how this mental illness compares and/or contrasts to other mental illnesses (e.g., depression, anxiety) or medical illnesses (e.g., diabetes, cancer).
- Ask the family to write a timeline of the development of schizophrenia in their loved one, together as a group project. Since the family will now be familiar with the causes of illness, they should be able to identify potential environmental and biological factors that may have contributed to their relative's illness. Encourage family members to take a curious rather than blaming approach to this task. In other words, try to ensure they do not point fingers at one another for having contributed to their loved one's stress.
- Related to the previous task, ask family members to sit down together and write out a timeline of the symptoms they noticed in

their loved one with the SSD (and potentially other symptoms that may have been missed) and of the steps they took to ameliorate their effects. Ask them to highlight the attributions they made regarding these symptoms. In particular, ask them to take note of negative symptoms (which are more likely to have gone unnoticed) or prodromal symptoms prior to an episode. In addition, ask them to note all their efforts to understand and ameliorate symptoms (i.e., who did they go to for help—medical doctor, priest, family, friends?).

- If applicable, ask the family to reflect on substance use patterns and potential alternative ways of recreating or engaging with others.

### Psychoeducation: Case Illustration

Juan and his mother, Maria, first heard about CIT-S during Spanish mass, when their priest informed the congregation about therapy available for mental illness. Juan's family had struggled for over two years trying to figure out what was causing the young man's odd behavior. After finding out that his diagnosis was schizophrenia, they tried to use every resource available. Following mass, they approached the priest to inquire about CIT-S. The priest spoke fondly of the clinician, with whom he had been working very closely, and said she was very knowledgeable about the important role that religion plays in well-being.

At 17, Juan had experienced a difficult break-up when his girlfriend cheated on him with his best friend. He felt humiliated, and because his ex-girlfriend and ex-best friend began dating, Juan felt he could not count on the support of any of his so-called friends. Moreover, he felt his family did not understand. His father, Miguel, told him to toughen up, and whenever Juan showed emotion, his father would say "*los hombres no lloran*" (men don't cry). Juan often missed school because he did not want to see his ex-girlfriend or ex-best friend. Whenever he did go, he would often cut class because he felt people were talking about the incident. During the weeks and months to follow, Juan became more and more isolated.

When Juan's parents acknowledged his behavior as a problem, they first took him to a *curandero* (healer). Both parents were immigrants from Mexico and although they have lived in the United States for over 20 years, they prefer to use folk healing practices, just as they had in Mexico, to deal with illness. After several months of bi-weekly visits to the *curandero*, Juan's behavior worsened and he began drinking heavily.

Next, his family decided that Juan should go to Alcoholics Anonymous, and although his drinking lessened, he continued to think that others were talking about him everywhere he went. He continued to miss school, was losing a lot of weight because he would not eat, and was frequently observed talking to himself. His parents then took him to a family doctor who referred them to psychiatry. Juan was diagnosed with schizophrenia at 19, two years after his symptoms began. Despite the diagnosis and the medication education they received, Miguel refused to give Juan the medication. Miguel hoped that as Juan matured and became an *hombre* (a man), his symptoms would stabilize. Months went by, and Juan's medication became a point of major conflict in his parents' marriage, with his mother, Maria, eager to give the medications a try. Juan's father eventually agreed that Juan should try medication, and after a few weeks, his symptoms began to lessen. A few weeks later, they heard about CIT-S from their priest at church.

After starting therapy, the family was pleased when they began to notice the changes in Juan's behavior. Everyone, including Miguel, began to believe that mental illness is something real and that it is treatable. While they could agree on this, some cultural values continued to interfere at the beginning of therapy. The primary concern was that Miguel did not trust the clinician because she was female. He had not been present at church when the priest discussed CIT-S; Miguel had assumed that the clinician would be male and was surprised to see otherwise. He openly questioned her ability to help his son, as he is a male. What Miguel did not initially disclose was that having a female clinician in an authoritative role was intimidating to him. The clinician anticipated that these types of concerns might be raised by families with more traditional backgrounds, such as Juan's, and Miguel's concerns were appeased as soon as therapy began, with the family collectivism module. Miguel's observation that the clinician was interested in their beliefs, culture, and family was new. After Juan turned 18, making him a decision-making adult by U.S. standards, it seemed to Miguel that doctors were no longer interested in involving him and his family in treatment. So, the fact that this therapy encouraged their participation and included an entire section dedicated to that topic made him very pleased with the treatment.

Within the psychoeducation module of CIT-S, the clinician described schizophrenia and explained the biopsychosocial model in detail. Following her description of the role that genetics play in the illness, Miguel noted that his own father had exhibited similar symptoms to Juan. He was treated by a *curandero* who lived in the neighboring town. The *curandero* explained that Juan's grandfather was *embrujado* (possessed) and treated him with folk remedies. His symptoms did not lessen, and Juan's grandfather died by suicide at age 40. This was a revelation to the rest of the family who knew nothing about this. During the remainder of session, they incorporated what they had learned in the family collectivism module and talked about the importance of maintaining harmony, as receiving this news was a shock to everyone. For homework, each member was asked to generate questions they had about the biological underpinnings of schizophrenia.

Miguel was eager to get started at the next session and opened with a prayer he had written in honor of his deceased father. His questions were about the prevalence of schizophrenia. Specifically, he wanted to know why his son had developed the illness when he, the father, had not. The clinician described evidence from twin and family studies to further elucidate the genetic literature. In addition, she spent more time talking about the psychological and social factors related to schizophrenia that were similarly implicated in the illness. These were discussed in the context of culture, and thus the family talked about *machismo* (masculine pride), the pressure on first-born sons to carry the family name, and stigma toward men with mental illness. The family began to realize that perhaps Juan's genetic vulnerability, coupled with the break-up and their pressure on him to toughen up, among other things, could have created a less-than-ideal situation where the illness was given a chance to develop. For homework, the family was assigned to consider how these topics (i.e., *machismo*) affect their current lives.

The third session of psychoeducation began with a prayer for Juan's continued well-being, which was written by Maria and read by Juan. The young man noted that while he was thinking through the homework assignment, he began to wonder what others thought of him. Juan reported that while he was doing relatively well, he sometimes felt like others were watching him, which made him worry that he was *volviendome loco* (becoming crazy) and made him question whether others in his community were afraid of him. The clinician began by guiding a discussion to explore the perceived meaning behind the word *loco*, and the family described that this word was associated with aberrant behavior, such as talking to oneself and with homelessness. However, what Juan meant when he used that word was his fear of becoming isolated, of believing that others were poisoning him, and of listening to the auditory hallucinations urging him to run away. Once the feared symptoms were described more specifically (and in a less stigmatizing manner), the discussion turned to relapse prevention. Knowing their history of medication noncompliance, the clinician talked to the family about the importance of medication to maintain stability. Given Juan's history of drinking, the group also talked about the importance of refraining from drinking despite this activity being common among the men in their family and community. For homework, the family was asked to write about what it means in their culture to be someone with a drinking problem versus someone with a serious mental illness.

By the end of this module, Juan and his family felt they had cleared up many of the misconceptions about his mental illness. They had uncovered family history that made them feel more united. The safe environment they created helped the family comfortably ask questions about mental illness and their culture. As therapy progressed, Juan's symptoms lessened, he received more emotional support and less criticism from his family, he and his family were better able to identify Juan's symptoms and recognize their incorrect attributions, and Juan began to expand his social support network.

# CHAPTER 5

# Module 3—Spirituality (Sessions 7–9)

## Handouts for This Module

Refer to Table 5.1 later in this chapter for suggestions on how to break the module into three sessions and which handout(s) to use for each session.

- Handout 9: Religion and Spirituality
- Handout 10: Existential and Philosophical Beliefs
- Handout 11: Spiritual Methods of Coping

## Background Information for the Clinician

Approximately 87% of Americans report that they believe in God (Gallup Poll, n.d.) and over half (55%) of adult Americans engage in daily prayer (Pew Research Center, 2018). This number is even higher for people with schizophrenia. In a study by Nolan and colleagues (2012), 91% of people with schizophrenia in the southeastern United States reported engaging in religious or spiritual (R/S) activities and 68% reported participation in public religious services and activities. Thus, religion and spirituality are significant components of many contemporary lives, including the lives of individuals with schizophrenia spectrum disorders (SSDs).

In many ways, the widespread prevalence of R/S in the United States is encouraging. Mounting research indicates that being R/S and engaging in religious forms of coping may improve mental and physical health. Religion has been found to be associated with multiple benefits such as delayed onset of physical conditions (e.g., coronary heart disease and hypertension); improved course and outcome of illness (e.g., reduced mortality after heart transplant and in breast cancer patients); and reduced rates of anxiety, depression, and substance dependence (for detailed reviews of this literature, see Koenig, Hays, George, Blazer, Larson, & Landerman, 1997; Koenig, Larson, & Weaver, 1998; George, Larson, Koenig, & McCullough, 2000; Payne, Bergin, Bielema, & Jenkins, 1991; Weisman de Mamani, Tuchman, & Duarte, 2010).

The mental health benefits of religion also appear to hold true for individuals with schizophrenia. Nolan and colleagues (2012) found that positive religious coping was associated with a higher perceived quality of life in individuals with schizophrenia. Similarly, in a sample of older adults (aged 55 plus) with schizophrenia, Cohen, Jimenez, and Mittal (2010) found that although religiousness was not significantly associated with psychotic symptoms, it did have a moderate effect on improved quality of life. In a more recent study, Das, Punnoose, Doval, and Nair (2018) found that individuals with schizophrenia, currently in remission, who used more religious and spiritual mechanisms of coping with stress, were better at planful problem-solving, positive reappraisal, and seeking social support from others. The authors concluded that a sound spiritual, religious, or personal belief system positively affects active and adaptive coping skills in people with schizophrenia, thus helping them cope more effectively with illness-related stressors.

With this data in mind, it seems important for mental health practitioners to capitalize on adaptive R/S beliefs and practices in the therapeutic process. In the spirituality phase of treatment, we aim to help participants tap into R/S and/or existential beliefs that may aid them in productively conceptualizing and coming to terms with mental illness. More generally, we aim to help them and their caregivers live more productive and satisfying lives. Correcting potentially destructive or maladaptive uses of religion is also a central aim of this module.

## Getting Started on Module 3

The duration of the spirituality phase is three sessions, and this module begins after the third session or upon the completion of the

Psychoeducation Module. It is important to note that the spirituality phase of treatment should be completed with all clients, regardless of religious orientation (or lack of religious orientation). You should reassure participants that it is not a goal of culturally informed therapy for schizophrenia (CIT-S) to steer them toward any religion but to improve the mental health and functioning of clients through whatever beliefs they may hold. There will be participants who report that they do not believe in God or who report that they believe in God but are uncomfortable or disinterested in a religiously based treatment. Assure participants that no attempts will be made to steer them toward adopting a religious stance. Instead of focusing on specific religious beliefs, clients who prefer a nonreligious intervention will complete similar exercises concentrating on their philosophical beliefs.

---

*Clinician Note*

*All handouts can be found in the appendix at the end of this therapist guide. You may photocopy the handouts for your clients, or you may download these items from the Treatments That Work Web site at www.oxfordclinincalpsych.com/CITS.*

---

## Introducing Module 3: Spirituality

Ask all family members whether or not they are religious and if they would like their religious or spiritual beliefs to be addressed directly in this segment of treatment. This will determine whether you give them Handout 9: Religion and Spirituality or Handout 10: Existential and Philosophical Beliefs. It is important to note that many questions posed on the Existential and Philosophical Beliefs handout are also relevant to clients who identify as religious and who choose to primarily work from the Religion and Spirituality handout. After distributing the appropriate handout, offer a rationale for the Spirituality Module, as some families may not see the direct benefits of discussing spirituality in therapy. For example, it can be helpful to acquaint family members with information presented earlier in this chapter (in the background section) indicating that having strong R/S beliefs and using religious forms of coping are associated with better physical and mental health.

This phase begins with a detailed spiritual history, which includes an exploration of each family member's spiritual beliefs and values. Handout 9: Religion and Spirituality and/or Handout 10: Existential and Philosophical Beliefs are useful tools in guiding this discussion. Encourage clients to discuss their beliefs (or disbeliefs) about God or another supreme being. Also ask them to discuss their notions of morality, including their beliefs about right and wrong and the meaning or purpose that they attribute to life.

Ask family members to outline their participation in spiritual or religious communities and to discuss any spiritual supports (e.g., priests, rabbis, imams) they currently have or would like to have in their lives. Also ask participants about spiritual practices (e.g., prayer, meditation, attending religious services) that they currently use or would consider using. Views that are commonly invoked for coping in many religions, such as God is always by one's side even in one's darkest hour, God loves everyone no matter what the circumstances, and God always has a higher purpose, even for mental illness, should be explored and encouraged if they are in line with the client's religious beliefs. Family members working from the Existential and Philosophical Beliefs handout should be prompted to discuss activities they partake in that represent their personal values (e.g., volunteer work) or activities that promote the values that they would like to engage in at a later date. Also encourage these participants to explore any meaningful mentors they have in their lives, or would like to have, who could help them bolster these values.

## Spiritual Coping and Shaping

Once each family member's spiritual beliefs and values have been explored, practices such as forgiveness, empathy, appreciation, and gratitude should be discussed. This conversation is best facilitated using Handout 11: Spiritual Methods of Coping. These values are at the heart of most religious traditions, and in our experience their importance is easily recognized by religious and secular clients alike. We encourage you to role play opportunities to increase these values among family members. For example, one client could express appreciation to another family member for the tasks they do at home (e.g., cooking, cleaning), and in response, the client on the receiving end could reciprocate by practicing the expression of gratitude for the praise. Teaching clients to respond with empathy and forgiveness toward one another (and others) is also an excellent way of attempting to lower high expressed emotion attitudes and improve the emotional climate of the household.

Research shows that experiencing and expressing all of these emotions (forgiveness, empathy, appreciation, and gratitude) reduces depression and anxiety (Bono, McCullough, & Root, 2008; Emmons & McCullough, 2003; Watkins, Uhder, & Pichinevskiy, 2015). Thus, frame role plays and other assignments aimed at increasing these values as ways of deriving the maximum benefits from one's spiritual/existential beliefs and practices. Encourage participants to practice these suggestions both inside and outside of the treatment setting in ways that may help promote practices of previous modules (collectivism, acceptance and understanding of SSD, etc.).

Other important exercises for this module should include having clients identify helpful R/S existential writings that appear relevant to coping with mental illness or to create their own passages. Encourage family members to bring these writings to session for discussion and to also read the material between sessions as a form of coping and self-help. Also encourage clients to engage in spiritual practices outside of treatment that they identify as personally relevant and potentially therapeutic (e.g., prayer and meditation) and to discuss these experiences in the following session. Ideally, these exercises/activities should be done as a family to increase a sense of collectivism and team spirit.

## Correcting Maladaptive Uses of Religion

As we have described in many of our published papers (e.g., Weisman, Rosales, Kymalainen, & Armesto, 2005), utilizing religion in psychotherapy is complicated and needs to be addressed with finesse. A fundamental issue that has kept R/S out of many psychotherapy interventions is the legitimate concern that R/S can sometimes be used maladaptively. During the Spirituality Module, you should reframe maladaptive uses of religion. For example, family members may express the belief that their loved one's mental illness is "God's punishment for some wrongdoing." This offers an opportunity to explore clients' perceptions of God and to help reshape pejorative critical views (which research suggests are associated with poor mental health; Ano & Vasconcelles, 2005; Harrison, Koenig, Hays, Eme-Akwari, & Pargament, 2001) into alternative, kinder, and merciful views. For example, this can be used as an opportunity to reshape the notion of illness as punishment and instead to view it as an opportunity to build character, virtue, and strength, which is in line with many religious proverbs: Allah does not burden a soul beyond what it can bear (Quran 2:286); for although the righteous fall seven times, they rise again (Proverbs 24:16). Another example is a client who passively turns to God to resolve their problems without attempting to take an active role in coping with life's adversities. For example, a client could report that rather than coming to therapy or taking their antipsychotic medications, they believe that "it is in God's hands" and just pray for assistance in managing their symptoms.

Organista and Muñoz (1996) have offered a few creative solutions that we utilize frequently in CIT-S, such as asking clients to share the exact content of their prayers. The authors reported (and we have also observed) that clients often state that they ask God to solve their problems. Additionally, Organista and Muñoz suggest helping clients to shift their prayers in a more active direction by drawing on popular sayings such as, "God helps those that help themselves." Other similar passages include "You yourselves must strive; the Buddhas only point the way" (Dhammapada 276) and "Allah will not change the condition of a people until they change what is in themselves" (Quran 13:11). This, they argue, can be used to reshape religious beliefs in a manner that encourages utilizing God and their faith to support and encourage an active and proactive stance toward illness management rather than a passive and receptive stance. You may also serve as a model for participants and ask them to recite prayers in which they ask God for support and courage in trying new behaviors. You can parallel other problems that clients may be more proactive in solving and do not leave in God's hands (i.e., finding employment or taking insulin for diabetes).

In a similar vein, exploring the ways in which God had previously answered prayers can be a useful exercise for shifting cognitions toward more active participation. For example, many clients resonate with the idea that God can answer prayers in subtle or indirect ways (e.g., a family member who suggests therapy or another helping coping resource). Thus, helping clients pinpoint instances where they were indirectly assisted by God can be a useful method for increasing self-efficacy (e.g., God helps those that help themselves). Furthermore, this approach can be used to increase feelings of gratitude and can help clients believe that they are not alone in their quest for illness recovery and self-improvement, as God is by their side.

Working with families who have disparities in their faiths can also present challenges. For example, some members may identify as R/S and choose to focus on their R/S beliefs in treatment, whereas others may not be religious or may prefer not to focus on their religion in treatment. In this case, give the religiously based handouts to the religious family members and the existentially based handouts to the nonreligious family members. Discussions with each family member as well as your suggestions and homework assignments should be concordant with each participant's orientation. Similarly, some family members may identify with one religion (e.g., Catholicism) whereas others may identify with a different religion (e.g., Judaism). Regardless of R/S orientation, all participants should be encouraged to respect one another's beliefs. Strongly establish this ground rule for therapy within the first session during the Family Collectivism Module of CIT-S and reinforce this throughout the intervention. It can be helpful to ask clients to explore shared values despite differences in R/S orientation. In practice, we have found that family members enjoy learning more about other members' religious and spiritual beliefs, even when they differ from their own, and this often brings the family closer together.

Finally, it is important to point out that we discourage clinicians from focusing on religion for families in which a person is identified as having religious delusions/hallucinations at baseline or anytime during the therapy. When this occurs, we instead suggest that during the Spirituality Module clinicians pose questions using the existential (i.e., nonreligious) handouts and discussion should be on more general constructs of gratitude, altruism, acceptance, forgiveness, and empathy, and the topic of religion should be avoided altogether throughout CIT-S. The rationale for this is discussed further in Chapter 8, where alternative considerations (such as working with highly symptomatic and delusional patients) are discussed.

## Dividing Module 3 Into Three Sessions

Table 5.1 is a guideline for how the three sessions can be divided in Module 3. As with all modules, some families will benefit from spending more time on one topic (e.g., spiritual methods of coping) than another or avoiding some topics altogether (e.g., the topic of religion for participants with religious delusions). Thus, we want to underscore that this is only an example of a session-by-session breakdown. We encourage you to adapt session content and flow based on clients' needs. It is important to note that each of the three sessions should begin with a prayer, followed by homework review, and end with a homework assignment from either the following list or another appropriate alternative.

## Additional Considerations and Conclusions

Upon completion of the Spirituality Module, participants should have a sense of how to adaptively utilize their spiritual and/or existential beliefs to come to terms with the hardships that often result from mental illness. Furthermore, family members will learn to exhibit respect toward other family members whose beliefs differ from their own, a habit that will build collectivism and reduce familial distress. Be careful to help clients with the SSD and their families channel their religious beliefs and religious coping mechanisms in productive and helpful ways and recognize when to focus on spirituality, existentialism, or a combination of both.

## Suggested Spirituality Homework Assignments

After having introduced the Spirituality Module and discussed whether clients identify as R/S, or would prefer to talk about existential/philosophical beliefs, for homework:

**Table 5.1 Sample Guidelines for Breaking Module 3 Into Three Sessions**

| Module 3 | Session 1 | Session 2 | Session 3 |
|---|---|---|---|
| Handouts | 9: Religion and Spirituality and/or | 10: Existential and Philosophical Beliefs | 11: Spiritual Methods of Coping |
| | 10: Existential and Philosophical Beliefs | 11: Spiritual Methods of Coping | |
| Content | Discuss the family's religious or spiritual traditions, practices, and beliefs | Discuss values that are most important to the family and how such values guide the family in determining what is right from what is wrong | Review R/S methods of coping and help the family identify R/S practices that will bring them peace and aid in illness recovery such as prayer, yoga, meditation |
| | Review R/S practices that have helped the family and others that may have caused them harm | Encourage values and practices that are adaptive (e.g., prayer), and help the family reframe or adapt those that are maladaptive (holding judgmental religious beliefs about the self or others) | Help the family identify R/S practices that they can engage in together such as singing hymns, attending religious services, or reading religious passages |

- Ask the family members to engage in their spiritual practices (e.g., going to religious services, praying) together, if possible. There should be a focus on those practices that have previously been helpful in coping with their difficulties. Family members should pay attention to any benefits (e.g., collectivism) that become apparent as a result of this practice so that they may be discussed.

- After clients have had at least one session of role-playing or discussing the religious notions of forgiveness, empathy, and appreciation, ask them to practice as many of these as possible at home. This will help foster a low-key, low expressed emotion atmosphere that will aid in the recovery process while also encouraging clients to engage in behaviors that likely align with their spiritual beliefs and values. Ask the family members to notice any differences that emerge as a result of this practice so that they may be discussed.

- Ask the family members to bring in spiritual (or philosophical) texts, parables, or materials that are relevant to coping with mental illness or family-related difficulties for the week so that they may be discussed.

- Ask the family members to reflect over the week about other ways in which they may use their spirituality to help them cope with their difficulties.

- Ask the family members to start a new practice that may be beneficial in the coping process or to increase the frequency of existing practices (e.g., daily recognition of things they are grateful for or knowing God is with them) so that they may increase the benefit they receive from their spirituality.

---

**Spirituality: Case Illustration**

Adam (44) and his son Ibrahim (21), originally from Egypt, attended CIT-S after Adam was attracted to advertisements that he saw online. Adam had been diagnosed with schizophrenia in his early 20s, soon after the birth of Ibrahim, his only child. While the pair had extended family living close by, father and son lived alone and mostly kept to themselves. Adam, who had been divorced for 12 years, was a devout Muslim who was very involved in the Islamic community in their city. He took a particular interest in CIT-S after learning that the treatment incorporated religious beliefs, which he saw as fundamental to his self-care and to managing his illness.

Adam and Ibrahim were seen by a male, non-Muslim therapist. Adam reported being relieved in some ways to be treated by someone who was not an integral member of the close-knit Muslim community, because he had concerns about privacy. On the other hand, he also expressed concerns that a non-Muslim may have difficulty understanding him and worried about being judged for his practices and beliefs. The clinician oriented Adam to the CIT-S approach to treatment, explaining how CIT-S incorporates each participant's religious views and explanations for illnesses and encourages them to practice their own beliefs and to heal through them. He said, "During therapy you will educate me about your beliefs, and I will respect them and use them to help you." Adam expressed a willingness to try it out.

Leading up to the Spirituality Module, CIT-S had been going well with the father and son pair. Adam was particularly receptive to starting therapy with a prayer and often brought Quranic verses to share. Ibrahim was also active, but while in the Psychoeducation Module, some conflicts between the pair had arisen when Ibrahim, a psychology major in college, wanted to emphasize the biological nature of the disorder while Adam expressed his views regarding the spiritual underpinnings of his experience. Adam believed that his first psychotic episode—which occurred while he was getting divorced and while Ibrahim was an infant—was caused by sorcery (which he referred to as black magic) that had been performed on him by his now ex-wife. He believed that this magic had sent a spiritual presence to his house that started to haunt him and eventually possessed him, leading to his illness. Ibrahim was less inclined to believe this version of events and backed his position by stating that every psychotic episode was closely tied to the mismanagement of medication on Adam's part. The clinician allowed for these feelings to be shared and hinted that these ideas would be revisited in the Spirituality Module.

The Spirituality Module was initiated by a discussion of the benefits that spirituality has on physical and mental health, with the clinician addressing areas such as meaning-making, social support, and alcohol and drug abuse. Adam and Ibrahim's spiritual histories were then explored by slowly moving through the questions in the handouts, with Adam choosing to work from the religious handout and Ibrahim choosing to work from the nonreligious handout. Both were given time to share their beliefs and values. Adam discussed how important Islam was to him. Our purpose in life was to serve Allah (God), who created everything. Adam lived his life according to the pillars of Islam by praying five times a day, fasting during the month of Ramadan, giving to charity, and even visiting Mecca (regarded by many as the holiest city in Islam) a few times in his life. When Ibrahim was able to drive him, Adam prayed at the mosque within the local Islamic center, and the sense of community there reinforced his religious beliefs and practices. He would often stay back after prayer to discuss his troubles with his imam (the person who leads prayers in a mosque), who often gave him advice on how to deal with day-to-day issues. Aside from his obligations as a Muslim, Adam would often speak to Allah directly via supplication (raising his hands). He would do this particularly in times of stress and felt that God was always there to hear him out. Adam believed that his illness came via Allah's permission and that only Allah could provide him with salvation from this life's worries.

Ibrahim stated that while he was raised Muslim and held onto many of the values that he aligned with, he had lost faith in religion over time. He no longer believed in an afterlife, stating that the idea "prevents people from living their only lives and perpetuates the injustices in this world." Ibrahim had started practicing yoga with his friends while also engaging in mindfulness meditation using an application on his phone. He claimed that his spiritual needs were met in this way. Ibrahim's beliefs were a source of distress for Adam, as it was his duty to raise his son to be a good Muslim. He thought that he would be answerable for Ibrahim's actions on the day of judgment. Son and father were requested (and agreed) to respect the other's beliefs throughout this process to reduce the anxiety between them while building family collectivism.

The clinician took this opportunity to reinforce the spiritual practices that both family members engaged in, reminding them of the many benefits as reported by research. The clinician even drew parallels between the two practices, noting how some poses in yoga and some forms of meditation are similar to Islamic prayer. He also shared the research indicating that individuals from developing countries often have better outcomes with disorders such as schizophrenia, lending more weight to the benefits of views such as Adam's. The pair were receptive, although Adam was keen to highlight how he is able to speak directly with God in prayer and felt that this was an important part of Islamic prayer that Ibrahim was lacking.

In the next session, the clinician gave out Handout 11: Spiritual Methods of Coping, which prompted the discussion and role-play of ideas such as forgiveness, empathy, appreciation, and peace. Both Adam and Ibrahim felt that forgiveness was an important value to have, and its benefits were discussed as they relate to an individual's well-being. They agreed that they should be more forgiving of each other's shortcomings and to consider that each is doing their best with the resources at hand. This was role-played by imagining a scenario in which one had wronged the other and going through the process of accepting what had happened and forgiving the other. Values such as appreciation and empathy were also role-played, with the pair taking time to appreciate each other and to convey empathy. Adam was a loving father, and despite his difficulties, he always did his best to make life easier for Ibrahim. His positive attitude and his efforts to overcome his condition were appreciated here. Ibrahim was his father's caregiver, and his important role was underlined while his significant efforts were reinforced. The clinician commended both of them for attending CIT-S and for their efforts in this module so far.

The discussion of peace revealed that Adam and Ibrahim do not argue often, and they attributed the peaceful environment in their home to Islamic values such as respecting one another. Both shared their views regarding Islam's role as the religion of peace, saying, "the word Islam means peace, after all." They shared the evidence that Palestinian Muslims have safely held the keys to churches in former Palestine for a thousand years, since Salahuddin took Jerusalem back. Adam also revealed how he grew up alongside Orthodox Christians in Egypt and that interreligious marriages were common. They felt that media and politicians had incorrectly been targeting Islam for the actions of a few bad people. They expressed how growing sentiment against Muslims was turning citizens against each other and was a source of great discomfort in their community. Adam also felt that Ibrahim was an atheist because he was afraid of being discriminated against. Ibrahim denied this, saying that it may be cultural and generational differences between himself and his father (who was raised in Egypt) that led him to adopt his own views. Ibrahim also stated that due to his obvious appearance as an Arab, he often still faces discrimination, irrespective of his personal views. Their insights were acknowledged by the clinician, who validated their experiences and empathized with them for the discrimination they faced. The four values of forgiveness, appreciation, empathy, and peace were framed as being integral to both Adam and Ibrahim's spiritual practices, and the clinician encouraged them to practice these values at home as well as in times of stress, such as when they face discrimination.

For homework, Adam and Ibrahim were assigned to continue their spiritual practices and to read and bring in some bibliotherapy for discussion.

### Clinician Note

*While it is normally encouraged for families to engage in the spiritual practice together to reinforce collectivism, Adam was uncomfortable with this aspect of the exercise due to his belief that mosques should only be a place of prayer to Allah. As a result, Adam and Ibrahim were assigned to practice individually and to read and bring excerpts from Islamic (or spiritual/scientific) scripture that were relevant to coping with mental illness or to the sessions thus far.*

During the third session, Adam had brought in some homework in the form of a Quranic verse that he wanted to start the session with. It read, "O My Devotees, who have committed excesses against their own selves, do not despair of the mercy of Allah. Surely, Allah forgives all sins. Indeed, He is the most Forgiving, the Merciful" (Quran 39:53). When questioned, Adam shared that he had been frustrated about Ibrahim's beliefs since the first session. Adam had spoken to his imam and was told that Allah forgives all sins, so the father should pray for his son with the knowledge that if Ibrahim wants to turn back to Islam at any point in his life, it would never be too late. The imam also reminded him that 113 out of the 114 chapters in the Quran start with a proclamation that Allah is the most gracious, and the most merciful. Despite a nagging anxiety regarding this issue, this led to some relief in Adam. The clinician circled the Quran's teachings back to the four points in Handout 11, which started with forgiveness. Then, Ibrahim shared some interesting research that he found regarding the benefits of religious or spiritual practices, stating, "These individuals have lower levels of depression and anxiety, and even live longer!" He agreed that his father's beliefs and practices may be conducive in dealing with schizophrenia and that forcing biological explanations for illnesses on his father may in fact push him away from therapy and be counterproductive.

The family's efforts throughout this module were reinforced by the clinician, who took this time to remind Adam and Ibrahim that his job was never to steer anyone toward a particular religious orientation but to encourage each individual to use their religious or spiritual coping mechanisms to heal. At the same time, the clinician reinforced the collectivistic view that both Adam and Ibrahim share the same goals when it comes to Adam's health. They spent a lot of time focusing on and caring for each other, and the mechanisms with which they undertake this process may be different but run parallel to each other. Adam and Ibrahim responded in agreement.

# CHAPTER 6

# Module 4 — Communication Training (Sessions 10–12)

## Handouts for this Module

Refer to Table 6.1 later in this chapter for suggestions on how to break the module into three sessions and which handout(s) to use for each session.

- Handout 12: Communication and Culture
- Handout 13: Expressing Positive Feelings
- Handout 14: Listening Attentively
- Handout 15: Making a Positive Request
- Handout 16: Expressing Specific Negative Feelings and Suggesting a Behavioral Change

## Background Information for the Clinician

Communication styles vary across ethnic and other cultural groups, and cultural beliefs and values implicitly and explicitly shape every aspect of the way we communicate within and outside of our families (Chesley & Fox, 2012; Dillon & McKenzie, 1998). Nonetheless, good communication skills seem to be an asset across most cultural groups (Dingemanse et al., 2015; Soliz, Thorson, & Rittenour, 2009), as research suggests that the ability to communicate and assert oneself appropriately are associated with better mental health (Berman, 2010; Speed, Goldstein, & Goldfried, 2018).

Communication problems can raise stress in any number of environments (e.g., work, school) including and, perhaps especially, within the family (Kymalainen & Weisman de Mamani, 2008). When a family member has a schizophrenia spectrum disorder (SSD), communication often requires extra effort because the symptoms themselves can cause the person to misread social cues in others, to convey thoughts in a confusing manner, or to avoid communication altogether by withdrawing from others (Bowie & Harvey, 2008; Möller, 2007). Not surprisingly, Merrill and colleagues (2017) found that communication impairment in people with schizophrenia is associated with poor performance in cognitive control domains, goal maintenance, and working memory and slower processing speed on automated tasks.

Unfortunately, communication is often impaired in the family members of people with SSDs as well. For example, communication deviance (CD), which refers to verbal transactions characterized by an inability to establish and maintain a shared focus of attention with a listener because of a lack of clarity or disruptions in speech, is often present at markedly higher rates in the family members of people with SSDs than in the general population (Miklowitz & Goldstein, 1997; Singer & Wynne, 1965, 1966). Interestingly, Kymalainen, Weisman, Rosales, and Armesto (2006) found that CD statements made by family members of different ethnicities tended to target different types of symptoms. For example, the CD statements made by White family members focused most on mental illness behaviors/symptoms that reflected a lack of independent functioning. For Hispanic, Latino/a, or Latinx and Black family members, however, CD statements focused most on mental illness symptoms/behaviors that interfered with the family's interdependent functioning. The authors offered data suggesting that the target of the CD comments reflected behaviors that were commonly valued in each respective ethnic group. Kymalainen and colleagues (2006) concluded their paper by suggesting that family members may have particular difficulty communicating clearly and coherently when discussing a loved one's symptoms that impact their ability to uphold important values and behaviors that are sanctioned by their ethnic background. We encourage clinicians to be mindful of this literature during culturally informed therapy for schizophrenia, particularly in the Communication Training Module. For a detailed review of the literature on CD and culture in families of people with schizophrenia, see Kymalainen and Weisman de Mamani (2008).

In the current module, we introduce a series of techniques aimed at helping family members communicate with one another in a clear, concise, and assertive yet civil manner. This approach will not only help individual family members to get their needs met but will also assist the family as a whole to maintain a low-key, low stress home environment. Many of the exercises and techniques in this module were based on a treatment first developed by Falloon and colleagues (1984) called *Family Care of Schizophrenia: A Problem-Solving Approach to the Treatment of Mental Illness* and a similar approach for bipolar disorder called *A Family-Focused Treatment Approach* (Miklowitz & Goldstein, 1997). We have adapted the exercises and supplemented them to make the techniques more relevant to people from diverse backgrounds.

In this module, role-playing serves as the primary technique to teach the communication skills in a nonjudgmental setting. One of the main goals in this module is teaching clients to speak to one another using the three Cs of communication: being *clear, concise*, and *confirming* what one hears. Another important goal is helping clients learn how to make requests for change from one another in a respectful manner that focuses on specific behaviors rather than on overarching personality traits.

## Getting Started on Module 4

Communication training lasts three sessions, and this module begins after Session 9, or the completion of the Spirituality Module.

> *Clinician Note*
>
> *All handouts can be found in the appendix at the end of this therapist guide. You may photocopy the handouts for your clients, or you may download these items from the Treatments That Work web site at www.oxfordclinincalpsych.com/CITS.*

## Introducing Module 4: Communication Training

Some families may view the introduction of communication training as carrying the implication that their communication patterns are dysfunctional. Offering families a clear rationale for the Communication Training Module will often help in this regard. You may introduce this section as follows:

> Now that you know a lot about schizophrenia and the symptoms, I'd like to begin talking about how to develop and maintain healthy communication patterns that can benefit all families with or without mental illness. In this module, our central aim is to help you develop a system of communicating with one another, and with others in your environment, that is in line with your values, will help you get your needs met, and will help increase the likelihood that your interactions are smoother and less heated. As noted in Module 2, low-key, soothing environments are not only best for keeping SSD symptoms at bay, they are also healthier in general and associated with less depression, anxiety, and stress.
>
> In this module, we will do a series of exercises called "role-playing." This means we will be asking you to turn your chairs to each other and practice new ways of talking among yourselves, such as praising each other, listening attentively, or asking someone to change their behavior. Throughout the module, we will ask you how this style of communication feels to you, and we will help you modify the techniques to fit with what is comfortable for you and in line with your cultural beliefs and values. We will also ask you to think about your values to help you decide which issues are most worthy of communication and which may be best ignored. In other words, one of the goals of this module is to help you pick your battles wisely and in a manner that reflects what is most important to you and your well-being.

## Role Plays

Role plays are at the heart of the Communication Training Module and will be the main approach for teaching and practicing communication skills. There are several steps in conducting role-play exercises:

1. Set the scene.
2. Model the skill for the participants.
3. Ask the participants to role-play the interchange.

4. Elicit feedback from all family members.
5. Model alternative ways of delivering the message.
6. Conduct new rehearsal with coaching.
7. Offer praise for efforts.
8. Highlight the proper application of skills.
9. Address areas of concern or improvement.
10. Give a homework assignment.

## Communication and Culture

Using Handout 12: Communication and Culture as a guide, this segment begins by exploring patterns of communication in clients' own ethnic or cultural background that may help or hinder them (e.g., indirect or deferential communication patterns; loud, boisterous exchanges). Family members are taught to think about their core beliefs and values when deciding whether to confront someone or make requests for change and to learn to pick their battles wisely. For example, sometimes it is better not to confront someone who makes an off-handed comment (e.g., a rude receptionist at one's dentist), especially if doing so would be considered disrespectful in one's own culture and would cause the person more distress or embarrassment than any benefit that might be gained. Instead, clients are occasionally encouraged to ignore small communication violations or problems and instead focus their energies on addressing issues that are of high importance in their value system and in their day-to-day lives (e.g., encouraging a spouse or child to communicate affection more often).

It is important to begin the module by asking clients to describe typical communication patterns in their family and culture of origin. For example, are some members (e.g., men, elders) expected to speak more often or more forcefully than other members? Is eye contact expected and an important part of communication in the family? Are direct questions common, or does the family utilize a more indirect form of communication? It is also important to ask clients whether there are topics or circumstances that are off limits for discussion in their family. This information can alert you to areas of discussion that should be avoided or addressed with caution. In some cases, explaining the rationale for why it is important to communicate about difficult topics can help to break down the barriers for discussing issues that you view as salient. For example,

> I know you have said that talking about money struggles is taboo in your culture, but we have found that many families dealing with an SSD struggle to pay for services and other things that could assist them with managing the illness. Thus, if you and your wife are able to communicate in session more clearly about where your different viewpoints lie about spending money and pinpoint what specific financial areas are most vexing to you, we may be able to use this information in the next module (problem-solving) to help you generate ideas for addressing these issues.

This discussion will also help highlight for you when it might be necessary to modify techniques so that you are not encouraging behaviors that could violate important cultural norms and cause clients more, rather than less, distress. For example, in some Native American (Thomason, 2012) and Asian (Leung & Boehnlein, 2005; Leong & Lee, 2006) cultures, direct eye contact with elders, bosses, teachers, parents, or other people in a position of respect may be considered disrespectful or rude. Thus, instructing clients to do so could be detrimental.

## Expressing Positive Feelings

Once you have discussed the family's typical style of communication and outlined their views on what would be their ideal approach to communicating, begin to discuss how to express positive feelings, using Handout 13: Expressing Positive Feelings. We find that it is helpful to begin with this topic, so that the segment starts on an optimistic note. Having family members turn to each other and offer praise or compliments defuses bad feelings, gives family members hope, and opens the door for more open communication about disturbing or conflictual matters.

The nature and purpose of learning to express positive feelings are to help make each family member feel valued and appreciated. We find that this approach makes family members more likely to want to continue saying nice things to one another and to engage in kind gestures, subsequently increasing family collectivism and team spirit. In introducing this skill, it is helpful to explain some of the components of Handout 13: Expressing Positive Feelings, to the family. For example, list the various ways to say "how it made you feel." Some people have trouble distinguishing feeling *good* from feeling *valued, relieved, appreciated,* or other emotions. Likewise, explain that this skill is for the purpose of offering praise for relatively specific behaviors of other family members; "You're a wonderful person" may not be as meaningful to a parent or spouse as "I appreciate how you've been helping me with the child-care." Then *model* the skill with one of the participating family members. Explain to clients that focusing on praising behaviors and qualities that are highly valued by the individual and the family's culture will likely have more of an impact than praising less salient ones. It can also be helpful to tie this in to earlier modules and remind clients that feeling and expressing appreciation, praise, and gratitude (toward self and others) generally helps people live in line with their religious and philosophical values and is associated with better mental health.

Once you have modeled the skill, help the family members *set the scene* by turning their chairs toward one another and talking directly to each other. One member is appointed the speaker role, and another is appointed to be the listener. Then, ask the dyad to *role-play the interchange.*

The process of modeling and rehearsing and then coaching by offering praise for positive performance or constructive feedback for areas of concern Is an iterative process, which is repeated through multiple role plays until the family member has mastered the skill. Then, ask the other family member (or members) to be speakers in similar role plays so that they too can practice expressing positive feelings.

## Attentive Listening

Next, Using Handout 14: Listening Attentively, you will introduce *attentive listening,* an essential building block for good communication. Family members coping with stressful challenges such as SSDs often have a great deal of trouble listening to the opinions, objections, feelings, or troubles of other members because they are often caught up in thinking about their own struggles. Moreover, cognitive deficits in attention may be a barrier. It is helpful to relay this information to clients and to further convey that learning to be attentive listeners and having a series of checks and balances to make sure one is listening attentively can greatly improve communication in families.

When introducing the skill, briefly discuss the difference between attentive listening and passive listening. Explain that attentive listening involves actively paying attention to what the speaker is saying and demonstrating this through body language (e.g., good eye contact) and follow-up questions and comments (e.g., asking related questions or reiterating what the speaker has said). During passive listening, on the other hand, the listener is often thinking more about their own response to the speaker's comment than to what the speaker is actually saying, and body language is disconnected (e.g., the listener may be looking away from the speaker and fail to confirm what they have heard). Thereafter, model the various components of attentive listening and solicit input from family members as to their understanding of and experiences with the skill. After modeling, ask the participants to attach labels (e.g., appropriate eye contact, paraphrasing, using nonverbal cues such as leaning in) to each of your listening behaviors. Then ask the family members to rehearse the new skill with each other, first regarding what appears (at least on the surface) to be a fairly neutral topic, such as discussing dinner plans or a television program that one member enjoys watching.

As was the case for delivering positive feedback, here you continue the iterative process of modeling, role-playing, providing feedback and coaching, and role-playing again (if necessary) until the family member demonstrates an approximation of the listening skill. Then, roles can be switched, and another member can serve as the attentive listener and the process can be repeated until each member has mastered the skill.

## Making Positive Requests for Change in Another Family Member

Using Handout 15: Making a Positive Request, the task of making positive requests for change in specific behaviors or actions of one or more family members can be discussed. When teaching positive requests, there are two specific components to keep in mind:

1. The request should be for another family member to *do* something, rather than to *stop* doing something.
2. It is not essential that the target of the request agree to do what is being asked. The request may be unrealistic or too difficult to perform, especially for someone dealing with residual symptoms of schizophrenia. However, once the family has completed the positive request exercises, you may help them resolve any remaining disagreements using the problem-solving approach in the next module.

You can introduce the positive-request section by stating to the client (Carol in this example),

> This next skill is called "making a positive request." As you can see in the handout, there are a few pieces to this skill: You look at a person, tell them what it is that you would like them to do, and say how it would make you feel. Carol, you have mentioned that you would like your husband to take you out on dates more often. How might you ask him to do that using this approach?

After introducing the topic, review the skill components. These are discussing the importance of having a clear goal in mind for the communication, framing requests with the "I" framework, and providing rationale for the request. Next, you model different ways to use the skill and elicit an example from the family that can be used to practice. Finally, as with previous skills, move on to role play and provide feedback during session.

## Expressing Negative Feelings About Specific Behaviors

In many ways, *expressing negative feelings* is the most difficult technique to learn. Unlike the other skills, it involves delivering an unpleasant, negative message. Nonetheless, this is important in that it offers family members a skill to use when making a positive request has been ineffective. Guide this section using Handout 16: Expressing Specific Negative Feelings and Suggesting a Behavioral Change. Specifically, this skill is a way of telling another family member in an assertive yet noncombative manner, that they are acting in an unpleasant or distasteful fashion. Assertive communication is confident yet polite and focuses on specific behaviors (e.g., "I would appreciate it if you would help with the dishes today. I have done them the last few days, so if you do them today I would be grateful as it would make me feel that our relationship is more balanced."). This is in contrast to combative communication, which is rude and generalized to the person rather than to the specific behavior that is causing distress (e.g., "You are a slob. I am not your maid, clean these dishes up now or else!").

As we noted in the background section of this module, communication is most likely to break down when discussing topics that violate cultural norms and practices (Kymalainen et al., 2006; Kymalainen & Weisman de Mamani, 2008). It is important to keep this in mind and to make sure that when clients are conveying their feelings, they are doing so clearly and that any instances of anger or communication deviance that occur are gently pointed out and corrected in the next role play. Helping clients gain insight into why a particular behavior is so distressing to others often increases willingness to change on the part of the message recipient and occasionally even deflates the negative emotion on the part of the message giver. An example might be helping a mother recognize that her daughter with an SSD who no longer wants to sing in the synagogue choir may not be rejecting her culture and faith but rather may be experiencing negative symptoms of avolition and apathy. The daughter's insight into the cultural and emotional significance of the mother's concern could enlist empathy on the daughter's part. Similarly, the recognition from the mother that the frustration really stemmed from her inaccurate fear—that her daughter was intentionally distancing herself from their culture—could help downgrade the mother's fear and the strength of the negative emotion, both of which are likely to smooth over their subsequent interactions about this topic and improve their revised role-plays.

As with previous skills, role playing is an effective approach to communicate the basic principles of this skill:

1. Look at the person; speak firmly.
2. Say exactly what they did that upset you.
3. Tell them how it made you feel.

4. Suggest how the person might prevent this from happening in the future.

You might say something to the effect of

> Esteban, you mentioned earlier that discussing money is difficult for you and your family, but you also said that your son's spending habits are causing a lot of distress in your family. Would you be willing to use this exercise to convey these feelings to Marco by telling him exactly how a recent spending behavior has upset you, how it made you feel, and how you would like him to behave in the future, so that this concern doesn't resurface?

As noted, expressing negative feelings can be the most challenging communication skill to teach in this module. Thus, family members often have to rehearse and role-play a few times before they can convey negative feelings in an assertive yet respectful manner that is likely to help them get their needs met. Thus, this technique should be role-played and rehearsed multiple times so that all family members can master it effectively.

## Dividing Module 4 Into Three Sessions

Table 6.1 is a guideline for how the three sessions can be divided in Module 4. As with all modules, some families will master certain tasks more easily than others. For example, for families who have good basic communication skills, the focus will be on more distressing topics where most people, with or without a mental illness, tend to have more difficulty communicating clearly. On the other hand, for participants with greater deficits in their communication skills, the attention will be on more basic skills such as making eye contact and paraphrasing what has been said before responding. Thus, we want to underscore that this is only an example of a session-by-session breakdown. We encourage you to adapt session content and flow based on clients' needs. It is important to note that each of the three sessions should begin with a prayer, followed by homework review, and end with a homework assignment from either the following list or another appropriate alternative.

**Table 6.1  Sample Guidelines for Breaking Module 4 Into Three Sessions**

| Module 4 | Session 1 | Session 2 | Session 3 |
|---|---|---|---|
| Handouts | 12: Communication and Culture | 14: Listening Attentively | 16: Expressing Specific Negative Feelings and Suggesting a Behavioral Change |
| | 13: Expressing Positive Feelings | 15: Making a Positive Request | |
| Content | Discuss the family's communication norms and review communication patterns that they believe are effective and others that they think could benefit from modification | Introduce the concepts associated with active listening and role play the skills | Discuss how to appropriately express negative feelings and make suggestions for the desired changes in behaviors |
| | Introduce the topic of expressing positive feelings and role play the exercise | Discuss the steps for appropriately making a positive request and role play the skills | Role-play the techniques for expressing specific negative feelings and suggesting behavioral changes in others |

## Additional Considerations and Conclusions

Even families or couples who formerly communicated well often have setbacks brought about by mental illness in a loved one. It is important to point out that good communication is one of the best ways to stimulate a healthy environment that is in line with one's cultural beliefs and values. If family members are able to employ good and respectful communication skills in the face of life stress, they will create a milieu that is more peaceful and potentially protective against psychiatric relapses.

In general, it is important to highlight that if individuals do not express their needs, they are less likely to be met. Moreover, communication skills take time to build. As such, they should be practiced as often as possible and incorporated into day-to-day life. Encourage clients not to become frustrated if difficulties arise, as this is common, especially as clients are mastering the skills, and instead, they can view challenges as opportunities to learn and grow.

## Suggested Communication Training Homework Assignments

After having introduced the Communication Training Module and the general framework of this approach, for homework:

- Ask families to write down some conversations they had over the week with members of their household. Have them write and reflect on these experiences during the week (e.g., How did they feel about the exchange? Did they tend to speak/listen more? Were their conversations calm or heated?) Use their reflections to jumpstart remaining questions about how culture/role influenced communication behaviors, praise aspects that are working, and explore areas that may need improvement.
- Choose a skill for the family members to practice during the week (e.g., attentive listening, making a positive request). Have them reflect on the difficulty, their comfort, and the impact (e.g., lowering expressed emotion, increasing perceived collectivism/family unity) of these methods of communication. This homework can be repeated as necessary.

- Ask the family members to reflect on conversations that were difficult for them or did not seem to go well. If a family member realizes they did not properly use one of the communication techniques, they can inform their family members that they want to redo the conversation and begin again with greater clarity.
- Have the family members discuss what thought distortions or thinking traps were clarified with effective communication practices. Moreover, ask what evidence was gathered to counter negative core beliefs they have.
- Have the family members practice some of the communication skills with people who are not in their family. Discuss how the experience and communication patterns differ when engaging with other people and in different contexts. Discuss how they may need to modify techniques when using them with people of different cultural backgrounds.

### Communication Training: Case Illustration

Christina and Destiny, two Black women, heard about culturally informed therapy for schizophrenia through their local church and were interested in attending with their adult son Xavier, also Black, who the couple adopted when he was 13 months of age. Xavier, now 23 years old, was originally diagnosed with schizophrenia when he was 18, during his first year of college. After his initial hospitalization, he dropped out of school and now struggles to maintain steady employment. He currently lives with his parents, Destiny, who is 50 and a social worker, and Christina, who is 55 and works as a travel agent. The couple met and began dating in their early 30s and adopted Xavier a little over a year after his birth in a closed adoption (i.e., no record of biological parents). Both parents are currently concerned about Xavier's long-term plans and his dependence on them. However, family members disagree on how to solve these issues.

Earlier modules solidified the family's commitment to one another and shared values. Christina and Destiny had been previously isolating themselves from their extended network and began to reach out again to grandparents, aunts, uncles, and cousins following what they learned in the Family Collectivism Module. Similarly, Xavier lost many friends as his illness worsened and he started to avoid communicating with them. He began interacting with some of his friends through online gaming and texting and then began inviting friends over to their home.

While both the parents and Xavier were frustrated that they did not know much about Xavier's biological family's medical history and how this may have contributed to his diagnosis, they were all encouraged by knowing that with proper maintenance, the disorder could be managed well. The Spirituality Module highlighted how the family used faith differently to manage their stressors. Xavier enjoyed his one-on-one relationship with God and felt empowered knowing he could seek God's guidance wherever he was. Christina valued foremost her faith community and the guidance they provided when she needed support. Destiny tended to focus on insights she could garner from scripture and prayer, which comforted her.

Working through each of the previous modules, however, family members reported that they had begun to communicate less and less to avoid conflict. Xavier noted throughout earlier sessions that since the onset of his symptoms he felt there was pressure on him to show he was doing well. It seemed whenever he discussed problems, his mothers ended up arguing with one another, which further reinforced the avoidance of communication. It was then during the Communication Training Module that the clinician asked each member to consider their patterns of communication and how their backgrounds informed their current communication habits.

Through this discussion, Destiny noted her discomfort with Christina's method of communication with Xavier. Destiny felt that Christina was too critical, focusing too much on what Xavier did wrong, and Destiny was worried this would lead him to withdraw. Destiny, having experienced a hostile and stern parent growing up, often felt like she had to defend Xavier from Christina. Christina, on the other hand, did not think she was being overtly critical, and she noted that Xavier was more likely to listen to her directions compared to Destiny. Christina's parenting, she noted, came directly from her mother and grandmother, who were straightforward and weren't afraid to hurt feelings if it's what their child needed to hear. In fact, Christina would have found it odd if her parents had not told her when an action was stupid or immature. In her eyes, these conversations kept her out of trouble and allowed her to mature. However, Christina also thought that her and Destiny's approaches could work in tandem. She joked that she felt she was the "God in the first testament" and that Xavier needed firm structure and foundation to survive, while she saw Destiny's role as "Jesus Christ in the second testament," quick to forgive and show mercy.

Xavier thought that avoiding communication was the only way he could establish some independence. When he was more communicative, his parents became more aware of his disorganized behavior, like when he lost his phone or forgot to go to work. When he was less communicative, they weren't aware of these problems, and he was able to solve the problem at his own pace. Xavier also liked to take long walks at night to clear his mind, but both Destiny and Christina thought this was too dangerous for him. After the onset of his symptoms, they especially began to worry that he might be more vulnerable, in particular if he came into contact with the police. Christina specifically noted that Xavier's poor social skills and forethought led him to wander into neighborhoods late at night. There had been two instances in which the police had been called and spoke to Xavier while he was wandering outside. This frustrated Xavier, who thought his mothers should see his ability to talk calmly to the police as a good example of his social skills. The clinician made sure to address how assertive yet noncombative communication may be beneficial to everyone's well-being and also would be useful so that Xavier would be more open to sharing when his symptoms were worsening. Noncombative communication would also help him think about how to talk to authority figures who could pose a threat to him.

The clinician asked the family members to keep their backgrounds in mind as they learned additional skills throughout the Communication Training Module. Some foundational skills such as being clear, concise, and confirming what one hears were introduced. Christina and Destiny noted that within their cultural upbringing, they were expected as children to confirm what their parents said, but parents rarely confirmed what their children said. While Christina and Destiny wanted to maintain their role as respected parents, they also wanted their conversations with Xavier to reflect his autonomy as an adult. For homework they were all asked to practice active listening with a particular emphasis on confirming what the other person said.

In the next session, the three clients noted that active listening was effective for the majority of the week. Xavier especially felt able to express his concerns and feelings when his parents took an active role in making sure they understood him. However, asking more questions and speaking frankly did incite more arguments. At one point, Christina commented on Xavier's lack of motivation to find a job, which prompted Destiny to argue with her on Xavier's behalf. During session, the clinician allowed the family to consider the effective and ineffective strategies of each member. Xavier stated that even though Destiny felt Christina was critical of him, he did not always feel that way. He felt he was able to comply with Christina more often than with Destiny because Christina was clear and concise. However, he acknowledged that when she asked too much of him, he rarely communicated this nor did he tell anyone he was struggling. Christina thought that while Destiny was a good listener, Christina was often unsure of what exactly Destiny wanted, which ultimately led to more fights when Destiny's needs weren't met. All members noted that the fighting that resulted led to greater stress and negative feelings.

To respond to this difficulty, the clinician transitioned into how to make a positive request. Bringing back skills learned from psychoeducation, the clinician asked Destiny to consider her thoughts, feelings, and behavior when she witnessed Christina confronting Xavier. While Destiny responded to the situation with an aim to protect Xavier, Christina, and their relationship, she acknowledged that this had not been the result. She stated that, regardless of whether she believed Christina's method was more hurtful long-term, Xavier was an adult who was capable of communicating his thought to his mothers directly, should he choose to do so. During session, Christina and Xavier role-played an argument they had earlier in the week without Destiny's involvement. All three clients used the handouts to address what went well and what could be improved. Christina and Xavier found it easy to offer solutions to each other, but they found it difficult to express their feelings, especially when they were both frustrated. The clinician highlighted this similarity and asked them to consider alternative options. Destiny suggested they could agree to pause the conversation and write down what they wanted to say through texts. Christina and Xavier agreed to try this method for homework. For homework, Destiny agreed not to get involved in Christina and Xavier's arguments and to explore whether this communication style reflected a role she liked to play in her family.

On the final day of the Communication Training Module, members noted their communication with each other had increased dramatically. Xavier, who was normally the quietest during sessions, notably led the group with his concerns. He noticed how communicating with his parents was improving their relationship, but he didn't want to fall into an unhealthy pattern again in which his mothers no longer treated him like an adult and constantly gave him directions. The clinician praised Xavier for using his communication skills to address a potential issue, and also noted that while the Communication Training Module was often used to deal with problems, similar techniques can be used to present positive information.

Using Handout 13: Expressing Positive Feelings, the clinician had the family members express positive feelings toward each other during session. Destiny led the group and commented that this type of communication came much more naturally to her, and she found that being direct and positive was much easier compared to when she had to express a negative feeling. Christina and Xavier, on the other hand, were less comfortable with the exercise. Christina thought her positive regard toward others was displayed through her actions and did not need to be explicitly said. Her family had not been verbally affectionate throughout her childhood, but she was confident of their love. Destiny said that while she understood Christina's viewpoint, she thought this was another skill that could be useful to Destiny's well-being. Xavier noted that while he liked the idea of it, he struggled to come up with what to say.

During the session, members attempted the exercise and compared how each approached the task. Destiny appreciated that Christina's way of expressing positive feelings was reflective of her personality: short, direct, and kind. Xavier, on the other hand, felt it was easier to think of concrete events, like being thankful for his mothers' cooking or for them spending time with him. All three said they would make an effort to balance the way they communicated with one another. The clinician then asked them to consider how their family had changed throughout treatment. While they acknowledged that their values remained the same, they were able to express them more freely and with less discord than they had before. They still had concerns about specific ongoing issues (e.g., Xavier's tendency to walk alone at night), but the clinician ensured them they had the skills necessary to approach these issues as they transitioned into the Module on Problem-Solving.

# CHAPTER 7

# Module 5—Problem-Solving (Sessions 13–15)

## Handouts for This Module

Refer to Table 7.1 later in this chapter for suggestions on how to break the module into three sessions and which handout(s) to use for each session.

- Handout 17: Problem-Solving and Culture
- Handout 18: Problem-Solving Overview
- Handout 19: Guided Problem-Solving

## Background Information for the Clinician

Surprisingly, the study of how culture influences problem-solving approaches has not received much attention in the literature. According to Güss and Tuason (2009), only 16 peer-reviewed articles from 1984 to 2008 were found on the topic. However, some research does indicate that different groups of people approach problems differently. One consistent finding seems to be how self-construal (members of a cultural group's propensity to be more individualistic or more collectivistic) influences how members of the group solve problems. As noted earlier in this clinician guide, people from more tradition-oriented and collectivistic cultures (e.g., Asian; Hispanic, Latino/a or Latinx cultures) are more likely to put group goals above their own goals when faced with life's problems (e.g., whether to take a job that is far from family), whereas others (e.g., White Americans and White Canadians) are more likely to focus on individual goals over group goals when prioritizing solutions to their problems (Radhakrishnan & Chan, 1997; Triandis, 1995/2018, 2001). Arieli and Sagiv (2018) further found that the likelihood of solving a problem was affected by the congruency between the problem in question (the type of thinking that is required to solve the problem) and the cultural mindset of individualism versus collectivism (the type of thinking activated by the cultural orientation). For instance, they found that members of an individualistic group (Jewish Americans) performed better on rule-based problems, whereas members of collectivistic groups (ultra-Orthodox Jews and Arabs from Israel) performed better on context-based problems. Thus, even within cultures, the type of problem may dictate the type of solution that is sought.

A study by Van Gundy, Howerton-Orcutt, and Mills (2015) examined associations between problem-solving approaches to coping with substance abuse on Black and White young adults and whether the effects of coping styles on substance misuse was moderated by race. The authors found that, for both groups, problem-focused coping (defined as attempts to alleviate stress directly by either changing the stress or the way one interacts with the stressor) was associated with reduced odds of illicit drug use disorder. However, Black young adults displayed less problem-focused coping and higher avoidance-oriented coping (defined as attempts to avoid or escape thoughts or emotions associated with a stressor) than did White young adults. Among White participants, avoidance-oriented coping was associated with increased odds of illicit drug use disorders. Among Black participants, however, avoidance-oriented coping was associated with lower odds of marijuana use disorder. The authors argue that there is an implicit bias assuming that avoidance-oriented approaches to solving dilemmas are inferior and that for some individuals and groups these strategies may be effective. Interestingly, while Black adolescents tend to have higher rates of stress exposure than White adolescents, Black young adults tend toward similar or lower rates of substance abuse disorder (Vogt, 2010). In short, although stress appears universal, how people cope with problems does not appear the same in all cultures. It is important to understand and appreciate clients' differing approaches to solving life's challenges and to help them maximize strategies that are in line with their principles and that are most likely to be effective for them.

The problem-solving segment of the treatment is concerned with teaching family members techniques to enhance their problem-solving capacities in ways that are in line with their cultural beliefs and values and that support their overarching life goals. As in the Communication Training Module, many of the problem-solving exercises in this module were drawn from other family therapies for serious mental illness (e.g., Falloon, Boyd, & McGill; 1984; Miklowitz & Goldstein, 1997) and adapted to be appropriate for families of diverse backgrounds.

## Getting Started on Module 5

The Problem-Solving Module lasts three sessions, and this module begins after Session 12 or the completion of the Communication Training Module.

> *Clinician Note*
>
> *All handouts can be found in the appendix at the end of this therapist guide. You may photocopy the handouts for your clients, or you may download these items from the Treatments That Work web site at www.oxfordclinincalpsych.com/CITS.*

## Introducing Module 5: Problem-Solving

The first step in this module is to offer the family a rationale for problem-solving. You can say,

> Up until now we've been talking mainly about how you communicate with each other. Now we would like to deal with some of the concrete problems of living that you have all been alluding to. But rather than just giving you suggestions about what to do, I'd like to teach you a way of solving problems cooperatively, as a family. Effective problem-solving is an important life skill that has been found to reduce some of the tension and family distress that develops in response to major life events, such as an episode of mental illness in a family member with a schizophrenia spectrum disorder.

Some participants may not initially see the relevance of examining and targeting their problem-solving approaches. In such cases, you may need to underscore the purpose of the Problem-Solving Module and discuss the fact that there is a strong literature base (e.g., Falloon, Boyd, &

McGill; 1984; Miklowitz & Goldstein, 1997) indicating that mastering problem-solving techniques can be a very useful skill in helping families with schizophrenia spectrum disorders to resolve their challenging problems. You may also have to assess the origin of their hesitancy. Some hesitancy in discussing specific types of problems may stem from cultural patterns such as viewing certain topics as taboo (e.g., sex) or certain contexts (e.g., mixed gender) as inappropriate for the discussion of sensitive topics. The next section offers guidance on exploring cultural problem-solving patterns in the family.

## Problem-Solving and Culture

As with communication training, it is important to take into account that culture influences problem-solving patterns. For example, some ethnic groups (e.g., White individuals) may be more inclined to discuss problems head on and to share feelings and emotions around difficult situations. Other ethnic groups (e.g., Asian; Hispanic, Latino/a or Latinx groups) may be more inclined to use a wait-and-listen approach to anticipate an appropriate compromise ahead of time. Throughout this Problem-Solving Module, it is important to discuss any cultural patterns or stances toward problem-solving and to work with the participants toward developing an approach that is comfortable and that works best for them and their family.

Using Handout 17: Problem-Solving and Culture to guide the session, this segment begins by exploring patterns of problem-solving in clients' own ethnic or cultural background that may help or hinder them (e.g., leaving problems to God, becoming hyperfocused on one aspect of a problem). You will also teach them to think about their beliefs and values and to use these to help them pick their battles wisely. For example, sometimes it is better to accept a lower-level issue (e.g., a family member who chooses to wear clothes to church that other members view as too casual), rather than labeling it as a problem. This is similar to many mindfulness-based interventions where a person is instructed to recognize a process or condition (often negative or uncomfortable) without attempting to modify or protest it. Accepting small problems can free up energy to focus instead on higher-level problems (e.g., a member of a devout family who refuses to go to religious services altogether).

Focusing our energies on problems that are both solvable and of high importance in one's own value systems can lead to a life that one can be proud of and that is both productive and fulfilling.

To hone problem-solving skills, it is helpful to begin by examining how clients and their family members, and/or other groups in which they frequently interact, typically solve problems. It is then useful to reflect on which of these strategies have been effective and which could be improved. As noted on the handout, families are then asked to ponder a series of questions such as "How do you decide whether a problem is within or outside of your control?" and "How do you decide what problems are or are not worth your time and energy?"

Once you have a clear sense of how the family typically attacks problems and which of their strategies have been perceived as effective/ineffective, it is time to present Handout 18: Problem-Solving Overview. You will orient the family to a set of techniques that help them (a) to identify problems, (b) to agree on their definition, (c) to brainstorm possible solutions, (d) to decide upon the optimal solution, and (e) to effectively implement the solution.

You can say something to the effect of

We think of solving problems as requiring a series of stages. These stages are a little like what we all do naturally in our heads, but there are some tricks to doing it as a family that make things go better. First, there is a definition phase, in which you try to identify what the problem really is and why it is a problem. This is a good place to reflect on your beliefs and values as a family to help you pinpoint exactly why something seems like a problem to you. Usually, the more specific you can be about defining the problem the better. Breaking the problem down into very small chunks can make it easier to address.

Then, as a family, I will encourage you to brainstorm as many possible solutions to the problem as you can, without evaluating any at that point. You will be asked to provide solutions that you view as viable and solutions that you don't believe are very good. It is helpful to have multiple solutions on the table and to thoroughly discuss the pros and cons of each. Discussing why "bad" solutions will not be effective often offers insights into what may make for a better solution.

Then, together, as a family, you will evaluate the pros and cons of each solution and pick one solution, or maybe a couple of them, that you think will work. Finally, I will have you discuss the specific plan you have in mind for implementing each solution. In other words, you will say exactly how you will put each solution into practice.

## The Problem-Solving Worksheet

Now that clients have had an overview of the module, give them Handout 19: Guided Problem-Solving and appoint one member of the family as secretary. It is often best to assign this task to either a family member who seems uninvolved in the discussions or, alternatively, to a verbose or tangential family member (including a symptomatic patient), as this puts more responsibility on that individual and increases the likelihood that the person will stay on task.

At this stage, ask the family members to identify a problem on which to practice the technique. We generally ask each person to suggest one problem that they think the family is currently facing. Although the family should have some say on which problem to tackle first, it is helpful to begin with simpler, concrete problems. As the clinician, you can help structure the problem-solving procedure by carefully guiding the family through the series of problem-solving steps, keeping them on task, and consistently praising them for their efforts.

If you encounter push back, first "take the blame" for the family's inability to solve the smaller problem they began with. *If it seems appropriate,* admit that you have encouraged them to solve a problem that is not really central to their concerns. Taking the blame removes the pressure from the participants and makes them less likely to feel like they have failed. When the problem-solving process is going well, offer guidance at each step and point out ways that might enhance the family's technique, but you should view yourself as more of a coach or a referee than a clinician. In other words, when problem-solving is going well, the family should be doing most of the work.

When the family is familiar with the problem-solving format, encourage them to generalize this skill to their home setting. For example, once the family has settled on a solution or set of solutions for a specific problem, you might say, "For homework you can carry out the solution plan and report back to me on how it goes next week. If it does not go well, we can come up with a revised plan, and if it does, together we can move on to a new problem."

You can also encourage clients to use skills they learned in earlier modules (e.g., communication training) when discussing problems. For example, participants may be able to practice attentive listening while other family members share their definitions of a problem, or they may practice making positive requests of other participants when generating solutions.

The final session of this module should focus on solving the specific problem of how family members can best continue to benefit from the techniques they have learned in culturally informed therapy for schizophrenia (CIT-S). Specifically, the session will address ways that families can increase the likelihood that they will continue to

1. Use one another as partners and support in the healing process. (See Modules 1: Family Collectivism and 2: Psychoeducation.)
2. Use the spiritual coping techniques learned in therapy to cope with life's challenges. (See Module 3: Spirituality.)
3. Pick their battles wisely and in a manner that is in line with their values and what matters most to them. (See Module 5: Problem-Solving.)
4. Utilize their new communication and problem-solving techniques after termination of the intervention to continue to function optimally. (See Modules 4: Communication Training and 5: Problem-Solving.)

## Dividing Module 5 Into Three Sessions

Table 7.1 is a guideline for how the three sessions can be divided in Module 5. As with all modules, some families will master certain tasks more easily than others. Similarly, some families will benefit from spending more time on one topic than another or avoiding some topics altogether. Thus, we want to underscore that this is only an example of a session-by-session breakdown. We encourage you to adapt session

**Table 7.1 Sample Guidelines for Breaking Module 5 Into Three Sessions**

| Module 5 | Session 1 | Session 2 | Session 3 |
|---|---|---|---|
| Handouts | 17: Problem-Solving and Culture<br><br>18: Problem-Solving Overview | 19: Guided Problem-Solving | 19: Guided Problem-Solving |
| Content | Discuss the family's typical patterns of solving problems and help them identify those that have been effective and those that have been ineffective<br><br>Give an overview of the problem-solving approach used in Module 5 and explain how this approach may help the family enhance the effective strategies they already use and how to overcome ineffective strategies they may have used in the past | Have the family identify a problem that they want to work on<br><br>Help the family operationalize the problem in their own words, brainstorm multiple potential solutions, discuss the advantages and disadvantages of each solution, and choose the best solution or best combination of solutions to practice for homework | Discuss the effectiveness of the previous week's problem solution and discuss how to further improve the strategy if needed<br><br>Select a new problem and have the family attempt to resolve the problem using the step-by-step guide presented in Handout 19 |

content and flow based on clients' needs. It is important to note that each of the three sessions should begin with a prayer, followed by homework review, and end with a homework assignment from either the following list or another appropriate alternative.

## Additional Considerations and Conclusions

This section of CIT-S provides families with a template for defining, generating, and implementing solutions to problems faced during their lives. In this module, it is vital to take into account that different cultures tackle problem-solving differently. It is therefore important to discuss any cultural patterns or stances toward problem-solving and to work with the participants to develop an approach that is comfortable and works best for them and their family. Teaching families how to solve problems as a family is a great way to build family cohesion and collectivism. It also decreases the likelihood that any one member will be blamed for family problems, as it shifts attention away from who is to blame for the problem and onto what can be done as a team to solve it.

## Suggested Problem-Solving Homework Assignments

After having introduced the Problem-Solving Module and the general framework of this approach, for homework:

- Ask the family to write a description of their problem-solving styles. Have them first think about and discuss their typical approach to problem-solving individual and family problems. Do they tend to harshly criticize each other, withdraw and remain silent, or do something in the middle? Does the family hierarchy and/or the family's cultural values and beliefs dictate whether or how problems are approached?
- Have clients block out a time to sit together as a family to discuss what types of problems are really worth tackling. Ask them to think about their values and how these play into what is viewed as problematic. Encourage them to select a few relatively small problems to

tackle first, which will help them understand the steps, before using these steps to address more salient problems.

- After clients have had at least one in-session practice tackling smaller problems together, for homework, ask them to sit together as a family to discuss recurring problems or more serious problems that they find troubling. Have them select one or two to tackle in session.
- After each problem-solving therapy session, have clients carry out the solutions agreed to in that session and prepare a narrative of how it goes (i.e., what works, what doesn't, and how the solution should be revised or retained in the future).
- Encourage clients to block out one hour or so per week, following therapy termination, to discuss individual and family problems and use Handout 19: Guided Problem-Solving to tackle them.

### Problem-Solving: Case Illustration

Jayne and her daughter Barbara first learned of CIT-S through family friends at a Bat Mitzvah. This family friend was a rabbi who had learned of CIT-S at a religious networking event. The rabbi knew that Jayne was diagnosed with schizophrenia and made a note to inform her of this resource the next time they met. Jayne and Barbara had been arguing a lot recently, and they had some friends who had attended therapy before and did not experience any improvement in their mental health. Nonetheless, the rabbi encouraged them to give CIT-S a try, and she explained that this treatment was different from traditional therapy because it incorporated topics concerning family and religion. Once they heard this, Jayne and Barbara became interested and started seeing their CIT-S therapist a couple weeks later.

Jayne had developed symptoms of schizophrenia following stressful and traumatic events. Her childhood and adolescence had been safe and fun. She married the love of her life at 20, and they became pregnant. Her husband suffered a fatal accident and died three months after they wed. Jayne was two months pregnant at the time and coping with all of this was proving extremely difficult. She began to hear voices during pregnancy, and her symptoms worsened after giving birth. She was diagnosed with schizophrenia at 23 years old; Barbara was two. For the next six years, Jayne had difficulty finding the right medication and adhering to it. She experienced multiple hospitalizations, and due to that instability, she was not able to consistently care for her young daughter. Eventually Barbara's custody was given to her aunt, Jayne's sister. This upbringing was difficult for Barbara and created difficulties trusting her mom for much of her childhood and adolescence. By age 30, Jayne's symptoms had remitted with the adherence of medication, and she was able to stay out of the hospital. Despite all this, Jayne remained a woman of strong Jewish faith throughout, and as such, she valued and deeply missed her daughter. Thus, she decided she needed to repair that relationship.

It took time for mother and daughter to build their relationship, but they succeeded and trust grew slowly and steadily over the years. Barbara became pregnant, and Jayne was very happy to hear that. In particular, she was excited to teach her granddaughter about Jewish culture and maintain it in the next generation. Terra, Barbara's daughter, soon became the center of everyone's attention and was loved by all. Terra, now 25 months old, was especially well-received by Jayne who saw her grandchild as a vital component of her life. However, disagreements started when Jayne's strong desire to be involved in Terra's life and Barbara's history of distrust for Jayne clashed. These arguments were their focus in the Problem-Solving Module.

During the first session of that module, Jayne and Barbara were given Handout 19: Guided Problem-Solving and were asked to focus on Step 1: What is the problem? Jayne reported that she wanted to babysit her granddaughter, but Barbara disapproved. In response, Barbara said that Jayne had "visiting rights" with Terra, as long as she, Barbara, was present. The clinician explored these statements further to get a broad picture of what each of them thought was wrong to arrive at one concise problem. Jayne connected this problem to her perceived role (as discussed in the Family Collectivism Module) as the "mentally ill" family member. Jayne instead wanted to be thought of as an independent, responsible, and caring grandmother, who was also a person who has a mental illness in remission. She had missed so much of Barbara's childhood and did not want the same to happen with Terra. Barbara, on the other hand, stated that she was unsure that Jayne could be trusted with Terra because she was worried that the illness would flare up given this added responsibility (as Barbara learned can happen in the Psychoeducation Module). Once the daughter and mother were able to recognize these perspectives, it was decided that the problem was that Jayne wanted to be trusted with the responsibility of babysitting Terra, but Barbara was not feeling ready to do that. While this was what they wrote on paper, they both understood that underlying this issue were very strong emotions of hurt and distrust. The remainder of session focused on brainstorming possible solutions to the problem using Step 2, the purpose of which is to come up with a list of many ideas. Their initial list included two items:

- Jayne visits Terra only while Barbara is present.
- Jayne babysits Terra all day while Barbara and her husband work.

These were very black-and-white ways of approaching the problem, and therefore the clinician asked them to generate more. So, they came up with a few more potential solutions, including

- Jayne takes Terra out for ice cream.
- Jayne and Barbara take Terra out for ice cream together.
- Jayne takes Terra out for a walk around the block, while Barbara is home.
- Jayne slowly works up to caring for Terra alone.

One of the key benefits in this module is that participants can generate several ideas that they may not have thought of before. We even encourage clients to list ideas that they think are "bad." Thus, the clinician continued to request potential solutions, and Jayne and Barbara added

- Jayne never sees Terra.
- Terra goes to live with Jayne.

Both Jayne and Barbara were reluctant to write down the last two options because they felt these were not solutions to their problem. However, the clinician noted that at Step 2, they were not to evaluate any of the possible solutions. Their task for this step was simply to generate ideas. He explained the importance of adhering to the chronological order of the steps now, while they were learning this approach. As they became more familiar with it, it would begin to feel more natural to do these steps in order. For homework, they were asked to complete Step 3, which is to evaluate advantages and disadvantages of each possible solution.

At the beginning of Session 2 of the Problem-Solving Module, both Barbara and Jayne were eager to find a solution. They asked the clinician what they should do. Kindly, he reminded them that this is their decision. The problem-solving handout is meant to help them visualize their options in a clear way; however, the decision would always be theirs to make and never the clinician's. He continued the session by reminding them that although this felt like a drawn-out process, it would be efficient in helping clarify all that was on their minds. Thus, the session moved to a discussion of their homework, which had been to list the advantages and disadvantages of each possible solution. They realized that many of their solutions had similar disadvantages. Thus, they focused instead on the advantages of each. In Step 4 (i.e., choose the best possible solution or solutions), they further realized that they did not have to limit their solution to one possibility. So, they chose a solution that incorporated three of those on their list:

- Jayne and Barbara take Terra out for ice cream together.
- Jayne takes Terra out for a walk around the block, while Barbara is home.
- Jayne slowly works up to caring for Terra alone.

Step 5, plan how to carry out their chosen solutions, was somewhat complicated for Jayne and Barbara since their solution was to be implemented over the span of a few months. They decided that Jayne would begin by visiting Terra only when Barbara was home, and they would occasionally take Terra out for ice cream together. After one month, if all went well, Jayne would then be able to take Terra out for an hour, for a walk around the block while Barbara is home, and after two months, she would be able to take Terra out for three hours at a time. Thus, they focused on the specifics of the first event in their more immediate action plan. For homework, their assignment was to implement the first step in their long-term solution: Jayne and

Barbara take Terra out for ice cream together. They were both to reflect on this experience and talk about it in the third session of the module, which was also the final session of the intervention.

At the beginning of the third session, Jayne and Barbara appeared excited. Jayne began by saying she had a very pleasant time with Barbara and Terra and that Barbara had even joined them for tea time. Likewise, Barbara reported that it was nice to have her mother around and to have her spend time with Terra. Step 6 is to review the implemented solution and to give positive feedback to all family members about their participation. Thus, the clinician attempted to further explore Jayne and Barbara's experiences in their first attempt at this. Jayne reported that she felt grateful that Barbara had allowed her in their lives. She confessed to feelings of guilt for having been in and out of the hospital while Barbara was a child. Jayne felt very strongly that children and grandchildren were her life's purpose, and she was grateful for that renewed sense of family. This was difficult for Barbara to hear, but she responded that, after having participated in CIT-S, she had a better understanding of the illness that Jayne had suffered with Barbara's whole life and the impact that her father's death and her own birth had had on her mother (i.e., the environmental stressors). Moreover, she told Jayne that she was proud of her for learning to manage her illness and that she had already noticed many strides at becoming more responsible over the past few months. The clinician praised them for their willingness to share such deep emotions and encouraged them to complete the remainder of the steps in the problem-solving handout in due time. This, he explained, would ease them into feeling comfortable with Jayne caring for Terra. Simultaneously, it would increase Jayne's sense of independence and responsibility, as well as increase Barbara's trust of Jayne. They also spent time talking about how to handle "hiccups" in their strategy. The clinician encouraged them to talk openly about things that could go wrong (e.g., Terra scraping her knee while under Jayne's care) and not to become discouraged if things did not go exactly as planned. The last and final step (Step 7) involved going back to Step 1 and trying a different approach if their plan proved unsuccessful.

"People often avoid making decisions out of fear of making a mistake. Actually, the failure to make decisions is one of life's biggest mistakes," Jayne said, quoting Rabbi Noah Weinberg. At the end of CIT-S, Jayne felt good about the added responsibility of and opportunity to spend more time with Terra; she had a newfound sense of independence and her role was shifting into more of a caregiver than a care recipient. She noted that she thought her daughter was beginning to trust her more and was hopeful that this trust would strengthen their family. Similarly, Barbara was happy to have learned more about the course of illness in schizophrenia; mainly, she was happy to consider that her mom may never relapse. She, too, was hopeful that her mother's illness would remain in control, that their arguments about Terra's care would dissipate, and that they would continue creating strong cross-generational bonds as a family.

# CHAPTER 8 ⟫ Additional Considerations

## Dealing With Unmedicated and Highly Symptomatic Clients and Clients With Delusional Thought Content

One important consideration is when a person with a schizophrenia spectrum disorder (SSD) may be experiencing symptoms too severely to benefit from culturally informed therapy for schizophrenia (CIT-S). In our CIT-S research, we generally exclude people who are unwilling or unable to undergo antipsychotic pharmacotherapy and those who we believe are displaying levels of psychosis too high to benefit from family psychotherapy. As discussed in Chapter 2, numerous double-blind, placebo-controlled studies in schizophrenia have confirmed the effectiveness of antipsychotic medication in reducing symptoms and increasing the intervals between relapses (Olivares, Sermon, Hemels, & Schreiner, 2013; Sharif, Bradford, Stroup, & Lieberman, 2007). Several empirical studies have also found that family-based treatment plus pharmacotherapy for schizophrenia are superior to pharmacotherapy alone (e.g., Dixon et al., 2010; Linden, Pyrkosch & Hundemer, 2008; Valencia, Fresan, Juárez, Escamilla, & Saracco, 2013). When psychosocial treatment is added to antipsychotic pharmacotherapy, there is evidence that relapse rates are reduced by as much as 50% compared with relapse associated with medication and standard care alone. Unfortunately, research indicates that people who are experiencing acute psychosis and are unmedicated do not benefit much from cognitive behavioral interventions or family therapy (Baier, 2010; Perivoliotis et al., 2010), as these approaches require a moderate degree of intact cognition to attend to and examine one's thoughts, feelings, and behaviors.

Given that CIT-S and other cognitive-behavioral therapy approaches ask clients to look for evidence to support their thoughts (Pervoliotis et al., 2010), those displaying exceedingly high levels of psychosis (which includes most clients with SSDs who are not taking antipsychotic medication) do not make good candidates for these approaches as, by definition, delusions and other psychotic symptoms are not rational and don't respond well to direct confrontation. For example, Zangrilli and colleagues (2014) found that when psychiatrists openly questioned delusional beliefs, this led to disagreements between the client and the clinician and put clients in a defensive position. In our experience, attempts to contradict or confront psychotic thought processes directly often have the unintended effect of reinforcing the delusional belief(s). Thus, when we consider clients to be experiencing symptoms too severely to benefit from CIT-S, we refer them first to medication management and encourage them to return when stabilized.

Because our clients are generally treated in the context of a research study, we have established clear criteria for designating when clients are displaying levels of psychosis too high to benefit from treatment. Specifically, if a client receives a rating of 6 or 7 on any of four core psychosis items on the Brief Psychiatric Rating Scale (Ventura et al., 1993) or if they are hospitalized primarily for psychiatric symptoms one month prior to presenting for treatment or any time during treatment, they are considered to be displaying levels of psychosis too high to benefit. As noted earlier, these clients are given referrals for medication management and encouraged to return when stabilized. In clinical practice, however, clinicians may be able to glean this information from a clinical interview. If a client is unable to hold a coherent conversation and stay on task for more than a few minutes or if their thought processes are so delusional that they will be resistant to approaches that attempt to examine and restructure maladaptive thoughts, they may not be suitable for CIT-S.

On the other hand, many clients with SSDs continue to experience low to moderate levels of psychosis and may still be able to benefit from CIT-S. For these clients (those who are not ruled out due to the previously described exclusion criteria), we attempt to carefully redirect the topic of therapy away from conversations that relate to the content of delusional thoughts. One common example is with respect to clients who experience religious delusions. Delusions of an R/S nature occur in nearly half of clients with schizophrenia, and clergy are often consulted by people with SSDs (Mohr, Brandt, Borras, Gilliéron, & Huguelet, 2006; Torrey,

1995). This is not surprising in that the onset of schizophrenia generally occurs around the same period of life when R/S and other philosophical beliefs are developing and changing. For this reason, it is not uncommon for R/S themes to be incorporated into a client's psychopathology.

As we have noted in earlier work (Weisman et al., 2005), when schizophrenia develops, many people with the illness experience intense heightened awareness and conclude that their R/S experiences (sometimes in the form of R/S delusions or hallucinations) indicate a special and unique relationship with God. As noted earlier in this chapter, in our view, CIT-S is only appropriate for clients who are currently medicated and not experiencing severe delusions. Thus, clients who have high degrees of religious delusions or hallucinations are not good candidates for CIT-S and should be referred out to a psychiatrist and stabilized on medication before enrolling in CIT-S. However, clients who experience low-to-moderate levels of religious delusions may still benefit from CIT-S. Nonetheless, it is important to emphasize that for these clients/families, a religious intervention may not be indicated. In our practice, if any family member expresses any degree of delusional thinking of a religious nature during CIT-S, the clinician is discouraged from discussing religion at all in treatment. Instead, the clinician targets philosophical and existential beliefs that are secular in nature (using the alternative handouts presented in Module 3) and opens and closes therapy sessions with self-help passages that may be spiritual but do not target religion directly.

## Dealing With Clinician–Client Concordance

What if clinicians do not share their client's beliefs and values? In Chapter 2 of this volume, we expressed the view that attempting to gain some broad knowledge of the history, philosophies, and typical customs of the primary ethnic, racial, and other cultural groups that we serve can be beneficial in connecting with and better understanding our clients. However, while research strongly shows that therapeutic alliance is one of the most robust predictors of psychotherapy outcomes (Borelli, Sohn, Wang, & Hong, 2019), it does not appear to be necessary nor beneficial for clinicians and clients to be matched on race/ethnicity and/or other cultural beliefs and values.

In our original treatment outcome study, which demonstrated the efficacy of CIT-S in reducing psychiatric symptoms in clients with schizophrenia (Weisman de Mamani et al., 2014), we also conducted secondary analyses to test whether treatment efficacy would be moderated by ethnicity and whether client–clinician ethnic match would relate to efficacy and client satisfaction with treatment. In line with our expectations, participants assigned to the CIT-S condition had significantly less severe psychiatric symptoms at treatment termination than did clients assigned to the psychoeducation-only condition. However, client ethnicity and client–clinician ethnic match (vs. mismatch) did not relate to treatment efficacy or to client satisfaction with the intervention. In other words, the treatment appears to work equally well for White individuals and minorities alike, and matching clinician and clients on race/ethnicity does not appear to impact efficacy. In another one of our CIT-S studies (Martinez de Andino, Brown, & Weisman de Mamani, 2018), we found that similarity between the clinician and clients in religious and collectivistic beliefs/values also had no impact on any therapeutic outcome variable, which extends the previously described findings. This finding is encouraging, as it is often difficult to match clinicians and clients in demographic characteristics and subjective values. Fortunately, the results of Weisman et al. (2014) and Martinez de Andino et al. (2018), along with other research (Propst, Ostrom, Watkins, & Mashburn, 1992; Rosmarin & Pirutinsky, 2020), suggest that the pairing of clinicians and clients regarding religious beliefs and other values may not be necessary to perform CIT-S and other cognitive-behavioral therapies effectively.

Interestingly, in a recent conference at the annual meeting of the Association for Behavioral and Cognitive Therapies, Rosmarin (2019) reported finding that in one of his recent studies, secular clinicians had greater efficacy than religious clinicians when treating religious clients. Thus, there may even be some benefit from not sharing clients' ethnic and religious backgrounds as clinicians may be less likely to make assumptions about how the clients may be thinking and feeling. To reiterate, we find the fact that clinician–client match on race/ethnicity/religion and other factors is not necessarily an asset is quite encouraging because it would be exceedingly difficult, if not impossible, to become an expert in the *culture* of all of the many types of clients that you are likely to treat during your career. Overall, in our experience, what seems to matter most in building a strong therapeutic alliance and in assisting our clients is a willingness and keen interest in getting to know our clients, as well as a deep respect for them and their cultural beliefs and values.

> *Clinician Note*
>
> *One note of caution is that whether or not you share your clients' ethnicity, religion, or other cultural beliefs and values, it is essential to examine your own cultural beliefs and values to make sure you are not imposing those on clients who may not share your values. To some degree, this is inevitable; therapeutic practice proposes changes to behavior and thoughts that could be cultural in nature. In addition, pointing out inconsistent or culturally inappropriate behavior can be extremely helpful and desired by clients. However, you should be reflective and should consider whether your comments/questions are made for the benefit of the client or are due to your own discomfort. Erring on the side of asking questions rather than providing advice/answers can help minimize this effect. To ground your practice, it can be helpful to remember that clients are coming because they are experiencing distress. Giving them necessary tools but being flexible to their point of reference can be useful in promoting change.*

## Dealing With Challenging Clients and Families

Let's face it, some clients/families are more challenging to work with than others. In this section, we describe some common challenges that we have experienced and discuss how we have dealt with them. One common challenge is when clients express doubt that certain treatment modules or exercises will be beneficial. When this occurs, clinicians should take a nondefensive stance and reiterate the purpose of the session and the exercises. You should also attempt to uncover any underlying issues that may relate to the hesitancy. The origins of the resistances often center on anger about events that have occurred, sadness over lost dreams and hopes, anxiety about social stigmas attached to the illness, and fears about the future.

To prevent or minimize the effects of denial/resistance, there are a few techniques you can employ. First, you can predict and anticipate these feelings with the family members when beginning each module. For example, in the Psychoeducation Module, this can be accomplished by acknowledging that coming to terms with a psychiatric disorder is a painful, confusing, and difficult process. Then you may explain to clients that these feelings are normal and that the therapeutic context is an ideal setting to discuss and come to terms with these feelings. You may also make analogies between medical disorders and schizophrenia, such as

> We can think of schizophrenia a lot like a medical illness, such as diabetes. People with diabetes also have a biochemical imbalance, only it's in their bodies' ability to use sugar. Without medication, in this case, insulin, people with diabetes can go into insulin shock and die. As a result, they need to learn to manage the disorder over time—become educated about it and its treatment and gradually accept it. The families must also come to terms with the fact that their loved ones have a chronic illness that requires ongoing care. This can create tension and conflict within the family. Perhaps what they experience is a little bit like what you are experiencing.

Another common challenge is dealing with clients who do not attend sessions regularly or who do not regularly complete their homework assignments. For clients who miss or reschedule frequently, we discuss with them whether this is the right time for therapy and if so, try to help them re-prioritize therapy. We explain that the treatment only works if it is regular and when the materials learned in session are practiced and reinforced between sessions.

We attempt to manage homework noncompliance proactively before it becomes a habit. When introducing CIT-S using Handout 1: Culturally Informed Therapy for Schizophrenia, discuss the importance of practicing the skills between sessions by completing the homework assignments and that homework is a critical factor in whether CIT-S will have a lasting impact. You might say

> Homework gives you an opportunity to come back with any difficulties you faced during the week so we can troubleshoot them in session. Research shows that individuals who complete their homework are better able to use and adapt these skills to make meaningful change in their lives.

One way to increase the likelihood that clients will complete homework assignments is to do a homework check-in within the first few minutes of each session. Keeping homework as a structured part of session encourages clients to come prepared. If clients do not complete an assignment, it is often helpful to have them complete it with your guidance in session, if possible. This reinforces the importance of homework, encourages practice, and allows the clinician and the client to assess obstacles that prevented participants from completing the assignment (e.g., did they have difficulty understanding it?). Another important consideration is whether the lack of homework completion is due to resistance or fear around doing the assignment. Processing with clients the reasons for noncompletion of homework and adjusting assignments accordingly are critical to increasing future compliance and progress in therapy. If homework completion does become a long-standing problem, using a problem-solving approach can be a helpful way for clients to increase their homework completion and practice CIT-S skills. For instance, if clients forget to do homework or run out of time during the week, they might pinpoint in advance when they will complete the assignment or consider reminders they could use (e.g., prompts on phone calendars, notes on refrigerators). You can begin subsequent sessions by quickly assessing the utility of these solutions and whether other approaches are necessary.

It is also common to encounter some hesitancy toward engaging in role-plays. In some cases, people may feel anxious or nervous regarding role-playing exercises because they may feel silly or awkward doing them or may feel they are unable to act convincingly. There are different ways to address this sort of concern, including allowing other family members to provide suggestions during the role-play interactions to help another member finish the point and arrive at the "correct" or appropriate solution. It is also helpful to emphasize to clients that while most people feel awkward engaging in role plays, there is a lot of empirical evidence to suggest that they are an excellent way to learn and practice new skills that can lead to lasting behavioral change (Lehman et al., 2004). Having the clinician first model the primary role of speaker or listener (depending on the task) when the exercises are introduced often helps participants feel more at ease and willing to try.

Finally, a more challenging problem that occasionally occurs is when one or more family members wishes to distance themselves from their relative with the SSD. This happens most often in couples where the well spouse may be considering separation or divorce. It is also not uncommon for siblings or parents who have sacrificed time and money attending to the person with an SSD to wish to diminish or discontinue in their caregiving role. One way to encourage such clients is to explain that during CIT-S, the person with the SSD and the family members will be mastering many concrete skills that will help them to better manage the person's symptoms and will likely help the person establish a higher degree of independence, thus reducing their reliance on other family members. Throughout CIT-S we also discuss and promote beliefs and values that motivate clients to love and care for one another, even in difficult times.

# CHAPTER 9

## Integrated CIT-S Illustration

### The Case of Gina and Chogan

Gina and Chogan, both 30 years old, are a mixed-race couple. Gina is White with Irish ancestry who was raised in Boston, Massachusetts. Chogan is Native American (Arapaho) and was raised in Wyoming, where they met while Gina was traveling the country with her friends. They remained in touch after taking a liking to each other, and Chogan moved to Boston a few months later to be with Gina. They have been married for eight years, since they were both 22. Gina reported that she was raised Catholic yet is not very involved in the church, citing some mistrust. She reported attending Sunday mass from time to time and engaging in religious activities with her family, whom she describes as religious. Chogan, on the other hand, was raised in the Arapaho Native American traditions and still practices many of their rituals. He occasionally attends church with Gina, and Gina has borrowed some beliefs and ritual practices from the Arapaho tradition. Gina has had a diagnosis of schizophrenia since she was 25.

Just before Gina turned 25, her best friend June went missing in the Boston winter. June's body was found three months later, after the snow had receded. Gina reported being very close to June's family throughout her life and more so during this period, sharing in their distress and organizing/leading local search parties that tried to locate June's whereabouts. It was during this stressful time that Gina first noticed that something was not right with her. She began feeling strange and started increasingly isolating herself from others and immersing herself in her search for June. Soon after June's body was discovered, Gina reported hearing whispering voices, as if June (or someone pretending to be June) was trying to speak with her, although the voices were mostly indiscernible. Gina also started believing that people who she encountered on the street were part of a large conspiracy to cover up June's murder, and that they were trying to implant ideas in her brain that would make it impossible for her to solve the crime. One day, Gina went missing and was found at night, walking barefoot on the roadside and speaking back to the whispering voices she was hearing. It was at this point that Gina's parents took her to see a psychiatrist.

Gina's psychiatrist diagnosed her with schizophrenia, prescribed antipsychotic medications, and recommended that she start seeing a clinician. One year later, Gina and Chogan moved to South Florida to escape the difficulties of winter in Boston, which also reminded her of the previous year's events and was impacting her treatment. It has now been five years since Gina and Chogan have been living in South Florida, where Chogan has a job at a casino and Gina is helping out one of her cousins with her thrift store. Gina reports finally having better control of her illness after a chaotic initial few years, although it has not been easy for her and Chogan. She states that while she still feels as if June and other spirits are trying to communicate with her, the medication quiets them and makes it easier for her to manage day-to-day things such as working for a few hours and doing some chores at home. Gina is given limited responsibility at work, but her role has steadily increased over time. She reports that she is pulling her own weight but faces some difficulty as she is often forgetful. Gina also has trouble communicating with others; she often draws incorrect conclusions or jumps from sentence to sentence without completing her initial thought.

Chogan reports that he does not mind the state that Gina is in. His upbringing taught him that Gina's experiences are spiritual in nature and are a result of June's attempts to communicate how much she misses Gina. Chogan also helps around the house and is very supportive. The couple report having a very positive marriage despite some difficulties with communication and rare psychotic episodes during which Gina usually ends up missing. Gina reports that she faces greater scrutiny from her own parents than from Chogan or his family, citing that she no longer opens up to her own family about the alternative treatments she has tried, such as aromatherapy, sage, and dreamwork. The couple heard about CIT-S from a friend who works at the thrift store. Gina and Chogan decided to try it out to help alleviate some of the distress in their lives and to provide coping strategies that address their cultural and spiritual nuances. They hope that if they are able to get a better handle on their difficulties, they can return to life in Boston where they can start a family.

## Module 1: Family Collectivism

### Family Collectivism 1—Week 1

The first session of CIT-S began with a nondenominational prayer of hope about what the future can bring and the will to fight for that future. Gina and Chogan were then oriented to CIT-S, with the clinician taking time to introduce the goals, format, and expectations involved in the therapy, guided by Handout 1: Culturally Informed Therapy for Schizophrenia. At a glance, the couple were particularly interested in the final three (Spirituality, Communication Training, and Problem-Solving) modules, as those modules involved issues that the couple had hoped would be touched upon in treatment. In this initial session, the clinician spent a few minutes on rapport building with the couple, by briefly asking questions about their religious beliefs and living situation. The clinician praised Chogan for attending the family-based therapy and reinforced the commitment to Gina and to their relationship that he showed by attending the therapy. The clinician then asked the couple what they hoped to gain from the therapy, and they restated their wish to return to Boston in the near future, once they thought they had the necessary tools to be able to readjust to life there. They felt as if they were not too far away from their goal. The clinician discussed wanting to keep that goal in mind as they progressed through the modules.

The couple was then introduced to Handout 2: Family Dynamics and was asked to think about what family and community means to them and how each of them identifies as members of their important networks, taking cultural context into account. Gina and Chogan stated that family means a lot to both of them but described different ways in which this is the case. Gina comes from a nuclear family background in which she and her brother lived at home with their parents, and other family members were moderately involved in their lives. She remembers uncles and grandparents telling her stories of their migration to the United States. Chogan is part of a larger tribe and had grown up around extended family, sharing joys and sorrows as they navigated life on the Wind River Indian Reservation in Wyoming.

The clinician asked the couple whether differences in their cultural backgrounds translated into differences in their own home when it came to how they both defined family and community. They reported having combined their families in a way. For example, Gina described adding to her social support by forging close relationships with many of Chogan's family members as well as her own extended relatives. Chogan stated that, by moving away, he was able to maintain important ties while also gaining some distance from family or tribe members who may have been a source of unwanted stress in his life. When growing up, both Gina and Chogan's social support networks were hierarchical and paternalistic, with conflicts often rising between the fathers (who were at the head of the family) and others. These conflicts traditionally revolved around house chores or school performances, and family members were all answerable to the heads of the family. However, the couple stated that their current home environment is characterized by less of a hierarchy. Although the structure remains one in which Chogan is the primary bread winner, his behavior is described as more casual and egalitarian.

The clinician reinforced the couple's participation in the session and their willingness to open up. For homework, Gina and Chogan were asked to think about their current roles and contributions in their families and communities and whether they are satisfied with them. They agreed to complete this assignment and were looking forward to the next session. The initial session was concluded with another nondenominational prayer, this time one of gratitude for family and meaningful connections, for clothes and shelter, and for food to eat, as others do not have such blessings. The clinician informed Gina and Chogan that they were more than welcome to bring their own prayers to the sessions. That would allow the clinician to reflect on the prayers with them and, in doing so, would facilitate benefit-finding from within their existing spiritual practices.

## Family Collectivism 2—Week 2

Session 2 began with a prayer of healing and well-being, which also asked for the strength to overcome illness and disease. The clinician welcomed back Gina and Chogan to CIT-S, and they were ready to get going. The couple reported doing the homework, with each taking turns describing their roles within their families and communities at large. Gina stated that she had always been the odd one out in her family, fulfilling her obligations toward household chores as the oldest child but spending as much time as possible with her friends outside the home. Her role within her biological family was always fleeting. Gina described being distant from her family members (with the exception of her mother), stating that she felt uncomfortable at home and did not spend much time there as a result. When asked why, Gina responded that her father had "anger issues" when she was younger and would take his anger out on the rest of the family members. However, she reported that things have changed for the better over time.

Gina described having found another family in Chogan's, one that was very supportive and encouraged more involvement on her part. She described her role in this family as playful exuberance, with her giving and receiving love and nurturance. Gina stated that she wished to be closer to, more involved with, and more playful around her biological family members but that their criticism of her behavior since she had developed schizophrenia often turned her away. The clinician discussed how achieving this goal could be workshopped in the Communication Training or Problem-Solving modules. The clinician commended Gina on her willingness to complete the homework and her self-awareness. At the same time, Gina was informed how her roles in both families necessarily impacted other members of the families and that being cognizant of how we influence, and are influenced by, others is helpful in improving our relationships. The clinician also took time to discuss cultural differences that Gina had noted in the way that both of her families functioned and how distance between family members was more common among White culture. Gina agreed and noted that her family dynamics always felt normal to her.

Chogan reported being the youngest of five siblings and stated that his role was often that of troublemaker at home. Despite that, his family always appreciated his unique way of thinking about things. He often found himself at the center of family arguments, assuming the role of mediator. In his community, he was given leadership positions to help him stay out of trouble. He reported being satisfied with his role growing up and that he missed being at home. Chogan maintains contact with his family and is up-to-date with their current affairs. The clinician highlighted Chogan's positive role within his networks, explaining what a source of strength an individual with such a role can be for those around them. Gina also agreed and said that Chogan's role as a level-headed leader translates to their relationship as well. Chogan stated that while there is always room for improvement, he is satisfied with where he is within his valued networks, and the clinician validated his feelings.

Gina and Chogan also described their contributions to the community where they currently live. The thrift store where Gina works also accepts donations and provides products at heavily discounted rates for those in need. A few times a year, the couple helps to organize large-scale donations to assist the needy. This was a great source of pride for them, and the clinician took a few moments to appreciate their efforts and encourage them to maintain this activity. The clinician also informed them about the physical and mental health benefits of meaningful connections with other people. Connections made through rewarding interpersonal exchanges, such as donating or helping those in need, were considered part of eudaimonic happiness (the notion that living in accordance with one's character and virtue leads to a good life), and facilitate meaning-making and self-realization. Gina and Chogan were receptive.

The clinician assigned the following week's homework: What are the roles of your different family members? Think about their roles and contributions within your family and the community at large. Should they be contributing more or differently? Session ended with a prayer for increasing positive impact on those around us, and for helping build strong connections with family members and loved ones. Gina and Chogan were reminded that they were more than welcome to bring their own prayers, particularly as this would provide an avenue for the exploration of their spiritual values and their benefits. The clinician told them that if they wished to engage in spiritual narratives or to discuss religious experiences in lieu of prayers, that was equally welcome. The couple responded that they would consider that for future sessions.

### Family Collectivism 3—Week 3

Session 3 began with a prayer for appreciation of what everyone is able to do, paying respect to each individual's personal battles and limitations. Gina and Chogan were ready for the third session, and Gina had completed her homework, although Chogan did not have time to get to it over the past week. The clinician reminded Chogan that the homework was designed to promote introspection and facil-itate the healing process. Chogan replied that he had been interested in completing it and would do better in the future. Gina discussed the roles of different family members, demonstrating a theme of Irish pride. Her mother was a stay-at-home mom, who also taught Sunday school. Gina reported a positive relationship with her mother, with whom she remains in contact. Gina stated that she looks up to her mother, who is a positive influence in her life. Gina described her father as being a stoic and strict man who spent much of his time working. She believes that her father's temper and desire to work long hours kept him at a distance from the rest of the family members and their community, even though everyone knew him. She wished that her father did more to reach out but conceded that he is "just not outgoing."

Gina reported that her brother seemed to get along better with their parents and had gone on to college while she only received her associate degree online. Gina believed that she should be doing more at this point in her life, but she feels restricted by her illness. Chogan stepped in and exclaimed that he thinks Gina is doing a great job at home and work and that he had never thought that she was a failure. Her feelings regarding the contrast between her own situation and her brother's success were further explored in the remainder of the session and were validated by the clinician. The complementary nature of the contributions that each family member has traditionally made to make the family unit work was highlighted here. A focus on the commonalities between the members, instead of on the differences, was at the center of the message. It was agreed that every small contribution counts as a success and should be thought of as such. The clinician explained that our thoughts about a situation impact our feelings and consequently our behaviors, and both Chogan and Gina appeared receptive to this information.

The couple was then asked to discuss what their ideal family and com-munity looked like. Both described a healthy and happy family, where everyone was together. The clinician emphasized and encouraged their collectivistic ideal and took time to share some of the many benefits that strong social support networks have. Examples such as improving the ability to cope with stressors, lowering cardiovascular risks (including blood pressure), and increasing self-esteem were touched upon. When asked how their current families compared to their ideal families, the couple described that they were not that far off. For homework, Gina was encouraged to keep track of the contributions that she made to those around her over the coming week. Anything, as small as helping someone out at work to taking care of their pet dog was considered fair game for this list, which was not assigned a limit. She agreed to participate, and the clinician asked Chogan to help by providing Gina with a diary and pen and periodically reminding her of the homework. Session was closed with a prayer for family, to increase familial support, and to protect one's family from harm.

## Module 2: Psychoeducation

### Psychoeducation 1—Week 4

Session 4 began with a prayer to open minds to other possibilities and truths, as we are always students of life. Gina had completed her assignment from the previous week, which was to log the contributions that she made to those around her, no matter how small. Her list was a page long and included, among other things, smiling at strangers, giving her dog a treat or a bath, and helping an older woman carry clothes from the thrift store to her car. The clinician commended Gina on her awareness of the benefits that a positive attitude can have on others and on one's own well-being. Gina also felt that composing this list had increased her belief in her contributions to those around her and to society in general. She was encouraged to continue contributing whenever it was possible for her, taking her own limitations into account. The clinician also encouraged the couple to continue engaging in the activities that they enjoyed as a family to increase their connection with each other and to build upon the strengths of their relationships.

The clinician then shifted the conversation toward the next module, Psychoeducation, touching upon the importance that psychoeducation plays in the treatment of most mental illnesses. The couple agreed, but also aired their grievances about the psychological, medical, and pharmaceutical industries, in particular by how financially driven they are.

118

The clinician allowed them to share their views and relayed how alternative viewpoints regarding the illness and its healing are also beneficial and would be explored in this module of CIT-S. On that note, the couple's own cultural conceptualizations of Gina's illness were first explored, which also served to build further trust with the clinician. Chogan reported that the Arapaho elders, with whom he consulted, described Gina's illness as stemming from her close relationship with June and as an expression of the sorrow of June's loss. It was thought that June would always remain with Gina, with her voice increasing and decreasing in volume as her spirit continued to exist in the world. According to Chogan, the illness was seen as a blessing, as its purpose was to assist the healing process and to give power to Gina. He only became aware of the impact that psychotherapy and medication can have on her illness in the months after Gina was released from the hospital.

Gina's conceptualization of her illness could be characterized as coming from multiple cultural sources. She resonated with the Arapaho explanation of her illness, particularly due to the ways in which her illness had manifested (i.e., hearing voices that may be June or those who meant June well/harm). Gina also explained that her education led her to believe in the biological explanations of her illness and in antipsychotic medications as the cure to her symptoms. Her Catholic and Irish roots taught her to believe in God and to always do the right thing and that good things would come to her as a result. Gina explained that her current views allowed her to pick and choose what worked for her at any given time. She reported having adopted some Arapaho beliefs, as the ways in which they treated their mentally ill greatly increased her levels of comfort when compared with how her own family perceived things. The medication had significantly helped her with controlling some of the symptoms that made her life difficult, and she reported significantly fewer psychotic episodes when she was taking her medication versus when she was not. The clinician appreciated the value that each explanation of Gina's illness brought to the table, and the clinician applauded Gina for adhering to her medication while holding onto her other beliefs, stating that religion and science can work in harmony. For homework, Gina and Chogan were asked to write down how Gina's extended family perceived her illness and her symptoms, based on past interactions with them. Session ended with a prayer for the wisdom to gain understanding regarding other perspectives, as each may have hidden benefits.

## Psychoeducation 2—Week 5

Session 5 began with a prayer for the acceptance of what is and for the strength to fight for what may be. The clinician mentioned that the homework from last week would be discussed over the course of the session and moved forward in the module. Session started with the clinician educating the couple regarding the positive and negative symptoms of schizophrenia and the different ways in which they manifest themselves across individuals and cultures, including the fact that Gina's communication difficulties are symptomatic of her illness. The clinician facilitated a discussion of the cognitive deficits in schizophrenia, which allowed the couple to discuss the memory impairment and social cognition difficulties that Gina often faced. Gina reported often being off the mark when it came to understanding what was being said to her. Once in a while, she felt as if the individual to whom she was speaking had acted egregiously toward her, which would throw off her mood. Chogan reported that this often occurred at home as well, but that he usually thought that those difficulties were part of Gina's illness and brushed them off. Gina also reported that others were sometimes unable to follow her in conversation and told her she did not always make sense.

Gina discussed her memory difficulties, citing that she often forgot to complete her tasks or to return items to where they belonged at work, but that the relaxed environment at work meant that she did not have to face any consequences for her difficulties. The clinician discussed the importance that relaxed environments and reduced performance expectations have when it comes to lowering stress levels and symptomology and also reinforced the couple's approaches to Gina's symptoms. The clinician presented the use of mnemonic devices and other memory aids such as writing important tasks down on a to-do list and checking it periodically throughout the day. The clinician then asked whether Gina's biological family viewed her difficulties in a similar manner, and she said that they did not. According to Gina (who referenced her homework), some family members felt that her illness was a direct result of her own bad behaviors, citing their religious beliefs. Her parents, too, often criticize her for what they perceive as shortcomings in her functioning that should no longer exist now that Gina is medicated, such as the low number of hours that she works or her forgetfulness.

Such critical and emotionally overinvolved attributions and attitudes (i.e., expressed emotion) that are related to a poorer outcome of schizophrenia were discussed at length with the couple, who were then able to ventilate their feelings. The clinician also described the impact that high expressed emotion environments have on an individual's thoughts, feelings, and behaviors. The couple was receptive, stating that her family's attitude was one of the reasons that drove Gina away from home as she was learning how to navigate her new life. Her acknowledgment of the harm that such attitudes had on her mental illness and her willingness to do something about it were reinforced by the clinician. The clinician also informed the couple that addressing these difficulties with Gina's family would be role-played in the Communication Training Module, and they appeared pleased to hear that. For homework, the couple was asked to come up with real-world examples of behaviors that others engage in that could be detrimental to Gina's illness. Session was terminated with a prayer for healing, self-understanding, and greater understanding from others.

### Psychoeducation 3—Week 6

Session 6 began with a prayer of strength in the face of adversity, against temptation, and against that which may cause us harm. The clinician welcomed the couple back to therapy and asked whether they had completed the homework, which they both had. Chogan started a discussion of behaviors that would be detrimental to Gina's mental health, citing the pop culture example of rapper Kanye West. He reported that Kanye appeared in an interview where he claimed that he was no longer taking his medications for his mental illness, news that was met by applause from the crowd. While Kanye immediately alerted them that this was not cause for celebration, he admitted going off his medication to nurture his creativity when making his latest album. The influence that Kanye has over millions of his fans and the possible negative consequences of nonadherence to medication were discussed in session, and the clinician commended Chogan for completing his homework.

Gina reported on a behavior that would be detrimental to her illness: substance use. She reported having been exposed to many drugs while growing up in Boston and to having partaken in them throughout her young adulthood leading up to her first psychotic episode. Additionally, in Arapaho culture, smoking peyote buttons and marijuana in pipes was common at social events. The drugs were often passed around to guests and were used to facilitate interactions, stimulate conversations, and invoke deep thought. After Gina's diagnosis, she reported reacting poorly to any form of substance use. While Arapaho guests who would visit their home would often express their wishes to smoke, the activity would be conducted outside the home and away from Gina. The clinician emphasized the importance of staying away from illicit substances, citing literature that connects substances, such as amphetamines, with increased relapse rates in schizophrenia. Chogan's role in the healing process was also highlighted by the clinician, who encouraged him to take further action to maintain a safe environment at home for Gina. The couple were both commended for their thoughtful responses to the assignment.

Using Handout 6: How Does Schizophrenia Develop? the clinician moved along in the Psychoeducation Module, addressing the etiology of schizophrenia, including the biological and genetic predispositions and the role of stressors and major life events in the onset of the illness. The impact of day-to-day stress on the course of illness was touched upon. In addition, the clinician emphasized how one person or one specific incident is not solely responsible for the onset of an individual's illness. A discussion ensued, as the couple believed that June's disappearance had single-handedly contributed to the onset of Gina's illness. The clinician explored this with the couple and agreed that what occurred with June may have been a key event. At the same time, Gina's family history was significant for mental illnesses, such as an uncle who had an unnamed mental illness and her father who was described as "ill-tempered and isolated." The possibility that a genetic predisposition always existed was presented to the couple, although the clinician did not linger much on this point. The couple appeared receptive.

The clinician discussed Handout 8: What Can the Family Do to Assist? with the couple, which addresses different strategies for what family members can do to help an individual with an SSD. Chogan agreed to take greater responsibility in making sure that Gina remained adherent to her medication and that their home environment was as safe and relaxed as possible. The couple's continuing efforts in creating a low-stress, relaxed environment at home and at work were appreciated here, with the clinician emphasizing how important this likely has been in helping Gina to take control of her symptoms over the last few years. They were encouraged to make every effort to maintain a similar environment if they returned to Boston, and they agreed. For homework, the couple were asked to think of one more way in which they could make the home or work environment slightly less stressful for Gina. Session was terminated with a prayer for greater self-awareness and self-acceptance, knowing that we are all imperfect, fallible, and only human.

## Module 3: Spirituality

### Spirituality 1—Week 7

Session 7 began with a prayer for increasing spiritual strength and for maximizing the benefits that can be acquired from spiritual practice. The clinician then began with a discussion of the previous week's homework, with the couple stating that, together, they had come up with one way of reducing Gina's stress at work. They had purchased and brought a pocket diary (with a pen) that Gina could use to immediately write down any assignments she was given. This would prevent her from losing track of the different tasks that she needed to complete. The clinician reinforced their ingenuity in coming up with this strategy and agreed that writing down tasks would most likely assist in reducing Gina's stress at work by preventing the mistakes that may follow due to lapses in memory. The clinician then turned toward the next module, Spirituality. The many benefits of religion and spirituality on health were touched upon, and the couple was very interested to hear about the research.

Gina and Chogan's spiritual beliefs and practices were then explored using Handout 9: Religion and Spirituality. Chogan reported coming from a Northern Arapaho (white sage people) background in which he was very exposed to the teachings and practices of his faith. He reported an emphasis on men learning to fight and hunt and women learning to prepare meals and clothing. Many rituals were performed to connect with ancestors and with other creatures who deserved credit for the blessings that were provided to the Arapaho. Death was seen as a normal part of life and was celebrated at organized events that were attended by hundreds. Pipe smoking, sage, dreamwork, and ritual dancing were also a part of Chogan's spiritual practice, although he did not describe himself as particularly religious.

Gina, on the other hand, described that she was raised devoutly Catholic in a religious Irish family, although she was not practicing as devoutly anymore. She reported that she often attended Sunday school and mass while growing up, as that was part and parcel of being in the Irish community. She reported that she still attends mass once in a while with her cousins and Chogan, such as on St. Patrick's Day, as that was always a family tradition for her. Gina stated that since meeting Chogan, she has adopted some Arapaho spiritual practices that she is attracted to and thinks could be a source of benefit, in particular dreamwork and ritual dancing. She restated that the Arapaho explanation of her illness resonated with her, as she still felt some kind of a spiritual connection to June that emerged in her dreamwork and in her auditory hallucinations. The clinician appreciated the couple for sharing their views and reinforced their efforts in practicing some form of spirituality irrespective of whether they strictly adhered to a religious dogma. For homework, the couple was asked to think about similarities and differences in their philosophical and existential beliefs. Session ended with a prayer for spirituality, for greater understanding that we are all passersby in this world who share a calling to connect with something greater than ourselves.

### Spirituality 2—Week 8

Session 8 began with a prayer for sacred balance, to find a place between the real and magical where one can exist in harmony with oneself and with other beings. The clinician turned to the couple for homework. Both Chogan and Gina reported sharing a few philosophical and existential beliefs, which they had touched base on with each other over the past week. Gina reported believing in God while Chogan did not, yet both of them believed in a power that existed in all living beings. They valued leaving a small carbon footprint on the planet and saving the fish, birds, and trees. It was important to both of them to treat all living beings with love and care. Their concepts of morality revolved around preventing harm to other living beings and killing only to feed oneself and one's family. Chogan's warrior upbringing led him to believe in killing also to protect his loved ones. They both felt strongly against consumerist society and believed that excess was causing great harm to the world. The clinician validated the couple's views about the world, including their experiences, values, and philosophies.

The clinician then discussed some values that came with being a highly spiritual individual, such as forgiveness, empathy, appreciation, and peace, using Handout 11: Spiritual Methods of Coping. The couple and clinician reflected upon each of these values and also role-played. Gina tended to blame herself for some aspects of her illness that were beyond her control, and this was role-played with Chogan. The clinician taught him how to help Gina reframe the difficulties she faced and how to empathize with her in those situations. Chogan's positive role in Gina's life was appreciated by both the clinician and Gina, and role playing was conducted to practice how to appreciate Chogan's day-to-day efforts.

Peace was a theme that resonated with both Gina and Chogan's spiritual practices. Despite Chogan's training as a warrior for his people, peaceful resolutions always took precedence over violent ones, and the couple role-played heated situations in which they can call upon peaceful spiritual thoughts. For homework, the pair was asked to bring a prayer or symbol to the next session that has been important in helping them cope with difficulties (for Gina, specifically ones that helped her cope with her illness). Session ended with a prayer for enhancing spirituality and acquiring characteristics such as forgiveness, empathy, appreciation, and peace.

## Spirituality 3—Week 9

The session began with a spiritual passage that Gina shared, which was a poem that she always invoked in remembrance of June. She reported that it had significantly helped her and continues to help her in dealing with June's loss. To keep June with her, Gina had the poem tattooed on her body. It reads as follows:

Do not stand at my grave and weep. I am not there, I do not sleep. I am a thousand winds that blow, I am the diamond glints on snow, I am the sunlight on the ripened grain. I am the gentle autumn rain. When you awaken in the morning's hush, I am the swift uplifting rush . . . of quiet birds in circled flight. I am the soft stars that shine at night. Do not think of me as gone—I am with you still, in each new dawn.[1]

The clinician took time to appreciate the depth and power of the poem that was so important to Gina. Her decision to share it was lauded, and the clinician asked Gina to share some of her feelings regarding the poem. Gina reported going back to it often, particularly after she spoke to June's parents, as it helped her feel as if there was a greater purpose in life than just life and death and that June lived on through all of the amazing things in the world. Gina reported feeling more positive and less stressed whenever she spent time meditating on the poem, which she considered a spiritual experience. The clinician reinforced Gina's spiritual practice and also related the benefits that Gina reported receiving from this meditation to benefits of spirituality such as hope, optimism, and a positive world view.

The clinician then moved on in the Spirituality Module and asked whether the couple thought there were any aspects of religious or spiritual practice they felt were not as positive for its adherents. The couple took issue with aspects of organized religion such as forced practices, pressure to think and behave in ways that are not true to oneself, and judging others. Gina, in particular, had feelings of mistrust toward the Catholic Church after several high-profile cases of sexual abuse had emerged in Boston. As a result, the frequency of her visits to church had decreased. Her extended family's perceptions of her illness as having been a result of her own behaviors also led to her disengagement from practicing with them. However, Gina reportedly felt more comfortable attending her cousin's progressively oriented church in Coral Gables and

---

[1] This poem is attributed to Mary Elizabeth Frye in 1932. Although our search yielded no information on copyright, it appears that Frye intended this poem for the public domain. In an interview (titled "A Poetic Journey") with Kelly Ryan of the Canadian Broadcasting Corporation (CBC), conducted in 2000, a 96-year-old Frye stated: "I thought [it] belonged to the world—it didn't belong to me. I still feel that way. . . . It was written out of love, for comfort—if I took money for it, it would lose its value . . . maybe I'm a nut."

has continued to practice there. Gina reported that, at one point, her mother also stated that Gina's illness may be a result of her moving away from the Catholic Church. Gina reported that she had not internalized those thoughts, but that it did not feel good to hear them. The clinician then discussed Gina's family's religious views with the couple. The clinician spent time reflecting on the advantages and disadvantages that Gina's family's religious practices have shown in her life, and Gina concluded that the benefits far outweighed the risks for her.

The clinician reminded the couple that it was not the purpose of CIT-S to push for any specific kind of religious practice but rather to foster each client's practice so that they may gain the most out of it. The couple was encouraged to use those aspects of their practice that they felt were personally relevant and potentially therapeutic, and the couple agreed. For homework, the couple was asked to engage in a spiritual practice of their choice, such as meditation, dreamwork, or ritual dancing. The clinician asked that they perform the practice together to foster collectivism and then to note what benefits they had felt in the immediate aftermath of engaging in their practice. Session ended with an Arapaho song that Chogan brought as part of his homework. The clinician shared his admiration for the song and asked what it meant to both Chogan and Gina. Gina reported that Chogan often sang to her when she was upset and that this was a great source of comfort for her. For Chogan, the song invoked memories of all past ancestors and helped to reconnect him to the universe. The clinician reinforced their practice and requested that an additional item or prayer be brought to the next session if the couple were interested in exploring their spirituality further.

## Module 4: Communication Training

### Communication Training 1—Week 10

Session 10 begins with a prayer that Gina brought, which is Native American (of Lakota origin):

> Teach me how to trust my heart, my mind, my intuition, my inner knowing, the senses of my body, the blessings of my spirit. Teach me to trust these things so that I may enter my Sacred Space and

love beyond fear, and thus walk in balance with the passing of each glorious sun.[2]

The clinician appreciated Gina for bringing another piece of spiritual literature, and they briefly explored the messages that Gina and Chogan received from this prayer. The clinician then asked the couple whether they had completed their homework, which they reported having done. They said that they had spent one night over the past week attending a drum circle, where they spent hours dancing together. They reported feeling as if their bond was strengthened as time passed, and as if God and, in Chogan's case, ancestors were watching and feeling them move, which felt validating for them. The clinician reinforced their practice and then moved on to the Communication Training Module.

The clinician began the module by discussing the importance of communication in solving and managing many of the day-to-day conflicts and emotions that families face, such as those that Gina faces with her mother and extended family. The clinician framed the discussion as indicative of them being a normal family experiencing higher levels of stress, as opposed to being a dysfunctional family. The clinician then explored communication styles in both Gina and Chogan's families and cultures, using Handout 12: Communication and Culture. Both of them reported coming from loud and boisterous backgrounds in the Irish and Arapaho. They both reported that scenes of shouting were common in their households and during gatherings and that fighting between siblings occurred often. At the same time, family bonds were reported as being very strong, which also meant that families were increasingly likely to be dealing with situations such as coming face to face with each other to express their emotions. The clinician explored behaviors that the couple felt were helping and behaviors they felt were hindering their ability to effectively communicate with each other.

The couple was then taught the first of four communication styles: expressing positive feelings, using Handout 13: Expressing

---

[2] To the best of our knowledge, no copyright information is available for this prayer, which appears to be shared by many Native tribes and is most often attributed to the Lakota people. This finding was corroborated in a correspondence with team members of a documentary film, *The Sacred Science*, who have shared this prayer on their web pages (https://www.thesacredscience.com/a-native-american-prayer-to-awaken-your-spirit/).

Positive Feelings. This discussion began by coming up with a list of positive feelings that can be expressed as opposed to just "good" or "thank you." Then, the clinician modeled the role play with Gina and Chogan by expressing positive feelings about certain things that they had been doing over the course of CIT-S. The clinician then asked the couple what they noticed regarding the communication and received responses such as good eye contact, assertiveness, and attentiveness. The couple then modeled the communication style with each other, and the clinician observed and gave feedback. The couple then engaged in a discussion of how their cultures may perceive such a communication style. Both stated that they were curious to see how it would play out. They predicted that while their extended families could find such focused compliments odd at first, the feelings would most likely be welcomed. The couple agreed to practice expressing positive feelings over the coming week. Session was terminated with a prayer for greater appreciation of others and for the ability to adequately communicate that appreciation.

### Communication Training 2—Week 11

Session 11 began with a prayer for the ability to be there for others, so that they may be there in return. The clinician asked the couple about their homework, and both described having found considerable success in expressing positive feelings. Gina reported trying it with her cousin and with others at work with whom she dealt on a daily basis. She stated that they noticed her praise immediately and were visibly pleased with her words. She remarked how such a simple statement can have such a marked effect on others, and the clinician reinforced her efforts. Chogan also reported attempting this at work and was similarly pleased with the response that others had to this communication style. The clinician took time to discuss the positive impacts that expressing positive feelings in a more mindful manner can have. These can be reflected in our mood or in our interactions with others in our lives.

The clinician then moved on in the Communication Training Module by discussing two communication styles using Handout 14: Listening Attentively and Handout 15: Making a Positive Request. The clinician took the time to model both skills and then asked the couple what it felt like to be at the receiving end of those communications. The couple was then tasked with role playing those communication styles with each other. Gina took that opportunity to make a positive request for change from Chogan, which was to aid her memory by writing down and reminding her of certain important tasks like appointments or meetings. Chogan also practiced listening attentively while Gina made this request.

The couple then asked the clinician to discuss Gina's communication difficulties, such as her inability to accurately gauge whether someone is upset with her or not. It was agreed that a better way to go about such situations could be by thinking about alternative reasons why an individual could be behaving the way they were, as opposed to reacting immediately. Chogan then made a positive request for change by asking Gina to always think of alternative reasons instead of reacting, so that she may avoid getting upset and letting an interaction ruin her mood. Gina agreed to attempt that. The clinician then asked Gina and Chogan to think about how to alter problematic relational patterns by communicating more clearly with each other and with other family members. For homework, the couple was asked to practice listening attentively and making positive requests for change over the coming week, logging whenever it was done and how it made them feel. Session was terminated with a prayer for increasing ability to attentively listen and to act upon the wishes of loved ones, so that we may foster a more harmonious home environment.

### Communication Training 3—Week 12

The final communication session began with a prayer for increasing our comfort with words, so that we may be able to use them in beneficial ways and to avoid harming others with them. The clinician asked the couple how their homework assignments from the previous week went, and the couple provided reviews from others. In particular, both Gina and Chogan reported having tried listening attentively and making positive requests for change at work, no matter how small the conversation or request was. They reported that over the past week they felt that their bonds with their coworkers had improved, now that they were expressing positive feelings, listening attentively, and making positive requests for change. The clinician commended them for their diligence in using the techniques learned in session outside of therapy and informed them how that is the way to make the most of their experience in CIT-S.

The clinician then went on to the final lesson in the Communication Training Module, using Handout 16: Expressing Specific Negative Feelings and Suggesting a Behavioral Change. The clinician first modeled this communication with the couple, and then asked the couple to practice with each other. The couple discussed that they did not necessarily have negative feelings to express to each other as they were both very understanding and had a strong relationship. The clinician engaged them further by asking whether they could remember what their last argument was about. Gina stated that she had been upset with Chogan because he worked longer hours than were required of him, whereas her work hours were much shorter. Similarly, Chogan remembered feeling upset when Gina mistook his suggestions for criticisms. The clinician identified underlying negative feelings of incompetence, and the couple agreed to work with that when expressing negative feelings to each other and making requests for change. The clinician facilitated the communications, giving feedback to both Gina and Chogan regarding whether they had engaged in all of the points listed in the handout.

After the couple had practiced expressing negative feelings, the clinician asked Chogan to pretend to be one of Gina's extended family members. This was done so that Gina may practice conveying her discontent at their perceptions of her illness as stemming from her own behaviors or her lack of religiosity. The clinician also had Chogan pretend to be Gina's parents, so that Gina may express negative feelings regarding their excessive criticism of her difficulties. They explored different words or phrases that may be used. The clinician also asked Gina for feedback regarding whether she felt ready to engage her family members in conversations regarding these issues by using the newly learned communication techniques. The couple appeared prepared. For homework, the couple was asked to complete another few role plays using the same handout they had discussed in session (Handout 16). Session ended with a prayer for the ability to communicate effectively, including the ability to listen to others who need to be heard and the ability to share feelings that need to be expressed.

### Problem-Solving 1—Week 13

Session 13 began with a prayer for greater family collectivism and stronger bonds. The clinician started the session by asking about the previous week's homework. Chogan and Gina reported that they had attempted the homework by expressing certain negative feelings to each other as they emerged and that they had felt benefits of the exercise. Gina also reported that she had attempted the different communication techniques with her mother and father over a video call session. She reported that her parents were receptive to her communications, particularly as she took time to first express positive feelings to them regarding their continued support. The clinician reinforced their efforts and took time to appreciate the courage that Gina demonstrated by speaking to her parents about something that was a source of stress for her.

Next, the clinician introduced the Problem-Solving Module and provided rationales for engaging in this part of the intervention. Gina and Chogan both appeared receptive and ready to engage. First, the clinician used Handout 17: Problem-Solving and Culture. Gina and Chogan were asked whether there are cultural nuances in the ways that their two families solve problems. They responded that Gina's family members often argue and engage in the "blame game" when attempting to solve problems. Chogan reported that problems are normally not discussed until they reach a boiling point, at which point the elders are normally brought in. For smaller problems, individuals are expected to take it up with each other, with backbiting strictly forbidden. The couple were then informed how the Problem-Solving Model that they were about to be taught in CIT-S would follow a more structured and objective approach. The clinician noted that this problem-solving approach is not necessarily better than their cultural norms, but it has its own strengths so that Gina and Chogan have an additional tool available to tackle any issues they are facing.

The couple was taught different phases in the problem-solving process, using Handout 18: Problem-Solving Overview. Namely, they talked about agreeing on the problem, suggesting possible solutions, discussing pros and cons, planning and carrying out a solution, praising efforts, and reviewing the effectiveness. The clinician taught the couple how to pick out a few small/easy problems and attempt to solve them, and then the clinician walked them through what each phase would look like.

The couple was then engaged in a few complete rounds of problem-solving, from definition to solution, using Handout 19: Guided Problem-Solving. Gina and Chogan were asked to bring in the previously taught communication strategies to use here, such as listening attentively and making positive requests for change. The clinician appreciated their attempts at combining lessons. For homework, Gina and Chogan were asked to work with Handout 19 at home. They were asked to fill it out for two or three small problems that they both would face over the coming week. Session was terminated with a prayer for patience in dealing with life's difficulties and for the objectivity to be able to analyze and effectively solve our problems.

### Problem-Solving 2—Week 14

Session 14 began with a prayer for the wisdom to pick battles carefully. The clinician asked the couple whether they had completed the homework assignment over the last week, and they responded that they had. They mentioned that they had faced issues with forgetting to take the dog out for a walk and with Gina forgetting to take medication. They mentioned how they were able to come up with definitions of the problems that helped them look at the problem differently and helped them to solve it better. The clinician walked through their solutions with them and acknowledged their efforts. The couple remarked how these were issues that could end up causing much more stress than warranted, given how small they were. The clinician touched upon the prayer that started that session and took a few moments to discuss with the couple how it is sometimes better to accept certain lower level problems for what they are to avoid greater stress. That way, less energy may be spent overall. This would also allow Gina to spend more time on the important and solvable conflicts. The couple was receptive.

The clinician then turned back to Handout 19: Guided Problem-Solving, this time asking the couple to think of a larger problem that they were hoping to solve. They selected the issue of planning for what to do should Gina have another serious psychotic episode. The couple then spent time trying to define this problem. They drew from materials discussed in Module 2 and discussed which symptoms would be cause for alarm and at what degree of severity. They decided they were most concerned with delusions and hallucinations, particularly if these should get in the way of Gina's job or their relationship, and they were less concerned with other symptoms like tangential communication patterns or forgetfulness. They brainstormed several solutions (consulting with her psychiatrist regarding a medication adjustment, reducing demands and expectations on Gina until she appeared stabilized, hospitalization, etc.). The clinician reinforced their efforts and acted as a referee in this exercise. Instead of selecting one solution, the couple decided it was best to develop a hierarchy of solutions that they would use from least intrusive (e.g., adjusting Gina's medications and reducing demands on her) to most intrusive (e.g., hospitalizing Gina). They reported feeling reassured to have a plan in place should the need arise, and they decided to hang the completed handout on the side of their refrigerator for safekeeping. For homework, the couple was asked to come up with one other major problem that they were dealing with and to complete Handout 19: Guided Problem-Solving to find ways that they may achieve resolution. Session was terminated with a prayer of patience and mutual understanding.

## Problem-Solving 3—Week 15

The final CIT-S session started with a prayer of growth and self-appreciation. For homework, the couple had completed Handout 19: Guided Problem-Solving, discussing their move back to Boston. They had come up with potential problems that could emerge, such as stress, forgetting to pack certain things, and dealing with family members when they returned. They also went into potential solutions to those problems that they could try out, one at a time. They reported feeling more prepared to make the move back to Boston after being able to predict and analyze the difficulties that are most likely to emerge. The clinician appreciated the progress the couple had made in CIT-S overall and over the course of this module in particular.

The theme of the final session was "How can Gina and Chogan continue to benefit from the techniques learned in CIT-S?" The couple was asked how they can continue using one another as partners in the healing process, how they can use the spiritual coping techniques learned in therapy, and how they can utilize their new communication and problem-solving techniques after termination. Gina and Chogan came up with strategies that they could use to continue implementing what they have learned in CIT-S. They felt adequately trained in the techniques of communication and problem-solving, although they were aware that further practice would improve them even more.

The clinician reminded Gina and Chogan to continue monitoring the limitations that Gina's illness may impose on her, so that the home environment continues to be one in which Gina can be as relaxed and stress-free as possible. The clinician commended Gina and Chogan for their progress in CIT-S; the couple thanked the clinician, and both Gina and Chogan reported a high degree of satisfaction with the treatment and with their progress. CIT-S ended with a prayer for ease in the journeys to come, whether on the road to recovery, moving across the country, or the journey of mutual growth and aging.

# Handouts

---

*Clinician Note*

*All handouts can be found in this appendix. You may photocopy the handouts for your clients, or you may download these items from the Treatments That Work Website at www.oxfordclinincalpsych.com/CITS.*

Handout 1: Culturally Informed Therapy for Schizophrenia

Handout 2: Family Dynamics

Handout 3: Schizophrenia in the Context of Culture

Handout 4: Symptoms of Schizophrenia

Handout 5: Other Common Mental Health Concerns

Handout 6: How Does Schizophrenia Develop?

Handout 7: Course of Schizophrenia

Handout 8: What Can the Family Do to Assist?

Handout 9: Religion and Spirituality

Handout 10: Existential and Philosophical Beliefs

Handout 11: Spiritual Methods of Coping

Handout 12: Communication and Culture

Handout 13: Expressing Positive Feelings

Handout 14: Listening Attentively

Handout 15: Making a Positive Request

Handout 16: Expressing Specific Negative Feelings and Suggesting a Behavioral Change

Handout 17: Problem-Solving and Culture

Handout 18: Problem-Solving Overview

Handout 19: Guided Problem-Solving

## Culturally Informed Therapy for Schizophrenia

### Welcome!

*Culturally Informed Therapy for Schizophrenia (CIT-S) is aimed at helping families better understand and cope with mental illness in a loved one.*

### Modules and Goals

- Module 1: Family Collectivism
  - Reduce tension in family relationships
  - Improve sense of cooperation and team spirit
- Module 2: Psychoeducation
  - Discuss the cultural conceptualization of schizophrenia
  - Increase understanding and acceptance of illness
- Module 3: Spirituality
  - Increase spiritual and philosophical coping resources based on existing beliefs
- Module 4: Communication Training
  - Improve your family's ability to communicate with one another in a respectful yet assertive fashion that is in line with your cultural beliefs and values
- Module 5: Problem-Solving
  - Assist family in developing helpful problem-solving strategies in line with your cultural beliefs, values, and goals

### Session Format

Each session will last approximately 60 minutes.

- Sessions will begin with an opening prayer, scripture, or mantra that a member of your family chooses or, in some cases, the clinician provides.
- Next, family members will be asked to discuss the previous week's homework assignment.
- Session content, dependent on module, will take up most of the session.
- The next homework assignment will be provided.
- Each session will end with a closing prayer, scripture, or mantra that a member of your family chooses or, in some cases, the clinician provides.

---

*The content and format of this handout were inspired by Miklowitz and Goldstein (1997, p. 95).*

## Family Dynamics

*The following are questions to help guide the discussion about your family's roles and structure.*

### Family

- What does the word *family* mean to you?
- What does it mean to you to identify as a member of your particular family?
- What is the structure of your family (e.g., Is there a hierarchy? Are there alliances or conflicts between certain members? Does one member tend to serve as spokesperson or moderator?)
- What values (e.g., humility, community, achievement) does your family hold?
- What cultural or ethnic traditions does your family enjoy doing together? What is the history behind those traditions?
- How does your family help each other/show that you care for each other (e.g., doing or buying things for them, emotional support)?

### Your Role in the Family

- How do you see your role(s) in the family (e.g., the mediator, the helper, the scapegoat, the breadwinner)?
- Are you satisfied with those roles?
- How do you contribute to your family?
- Do you think you could or should be contributing more or differently?

### The Role of Others in Your Family

- What is the role of other members in your family (discuss each person)?
- How do they contribute to the family?
- Do you think they could or should be contributing more or differently?

### Family Goals

- What is your ideal family?
- How does your actual family compare to your ideal family?
- What steps or changes would be necessary to bring you closer to your ideal family? [*These are areas that we will continue to address in subsequent modules such as communication training and problem-solving.*]

## Schizophrenia in the Context of Culture

*The following are questions to help guide discussion about schizophrenia in the context of culture.*

- How is schizophrenia viewed within your culture of origin?
- What are the stigmas (if any) associated with mental illness?
- What does your culture of origin view as effective routes to the treatment of schizophrenia?
- How are mainstream approaches viewed in your culture of origin?
    - For example, is antipsychotic medication thought to be effective?
    - What about psychotherapy or family therapy?

*As noted on p. 19, the Psychoeducational Module was heavily influenced by earlier family treatments for schizophrenia (Falloon et al., 1984, pp. 178–204) and bipolar disorder (Goldstein & Miklowitz, 1997, pp. 87–185).*

## Symptoms of Schizophrenia

*Becoming familiar with the symptoms of schizophrenia is helpful in that it may reduce stress and you may become better able to identify signs of relapse.*

### Common Positive Symptoms (Behavioral Excesses)

- Hallucinations (e.g., hearing or seeing things that others cannot hear or see)
- Delusions (e.g., thoughts that most others in your culture would regard as unlikely)
- Odd thinking and speech (e.g., vague, metaphorical, overelaborate speech)
- Suspiciousness or paranoid ideation (e.g., beliefs that others are trying to harm you)
- Ideas of reference (e.g., beliefs that others are talking about you)
- Inappropriate affect (e.g., laughing for no reason or upon hearing sad news)

### Common Negative Symptoms (Behavioral Deficits)

- Constricted or flat affect (e.g., restricted smiling or facial expression)
- Poor hygiene (e.g., failing to bathe, wearing wrinkled clothing)
- Poverty of thoughts (e.g., difficulty finding words to express oneself)
- Slowness of movement
- Lack of motivation or drive, disinterest in close friends or confidants

### Common Cognitive Symptoms

- Disorganized thinking (e.g., thought pattern is disorganized)
- Difficulty concentrating (e.g., difficulty following instructions, planning)
- Memory impairments (e.g., managing information in the brain)

*The content and format of this handout were inspired by Miklowitz and Goldstein (1997, p. 100).*

## Other Common Mental Health Concerns

*It is common for family members, friends, and individuals with schizophrenia to experience other mental health concerns.*

### Symptoms of Depression

- Persistent sad, anxious, or empty mood (e.g., loss of enjoyment in activities you used to enjoy)
- Sleep disturbances (e.g., sleeping too much or having difficulties getting to sleep or staying asleep)
- Appetite disturbances (e.g., loss or increase in appetite)
- Feelings of worthlessness or hopelessness (e.g., feeling hopeless about yourself, your situation, or the future)
- Decreased interest in sex
- Poor concentration (e.g., trouble making decisions and/or focusing on everyday tasks)
- Thoughts of suicide or suicide attempts

### Symptoms of Anxiety

- Excessive and uncontrollable worry
- Restlessness (e.g., feeling keyed up, on edge, and unable to relax)
- Physical tension
- Sleep disturbances (e.g., having difficulties falling asleep or maintaining sleep)
- Poor concentration (e.g., having difficulties making decisions, difficulties concentrating on reading a book or on day-to-day tasks)
- Irritability (e.g., becoming easily angered or annoyed)
- Feeling tired or exhausted easily
- Feelings of panic (e.g., racing heart, sweating, shortness of breath, chest pain, nausea, fear of dying)

## Symptoms of Stress

- Poor concentration (e.g., having difficulties making decisions, difficulties concentrating on reading a book or on day-to-day tasks)
- Irritability (e.g., becoming easily angered or annoyed)
- Feeling tired or exhausted easily
- Sleep disturbances (e.g., having difficulties falling asleep or maintaining sleep)
- Restlessness (e.g., feeling keyed up, on edge, and unable to relax)
- Feeling blue, down, or hopeless
- Withdrawal from others
- Physical complaints (e.g., headaches, frequent colds, digestive problems, aches/pains)

## How Does Schizophrenia Develop?

*The emergence of schizophrenia is often misunderstood. The following are some facts about its development.*

- Genetic predisposition
  - The rate of schizophrenia in first-degree relatives of people with schizophrenia is 8% to 10% higher than that in people who do not have first-degree relatives.
- Biological predisposition
  - The nervous system may respond more strongly than it should, especially when under stress.
- Interactions
  - A stressful environment (e.g., increases in demands, life-changing events, sleep deprivation) may heighten the existing genetic/biological vulnerability.
    - In fact, age of onset for schizophrenia is usually in the late teens, when individuals are going through potentially stressful changes, such as beginning college or starting a career (stress occurs even if the changes are perceived as positive).
  - Drug abuse (e.g., alcohol, cannabis, synthetic drugs, cocaine) can also heighten the existing genetic/biological vulnerability

*The content and format of this handout were inspired by Miklowitz and Goldstein (1997, p. 120).*

## Course of Schizophrenia

*There is not a universal course for schizophrenia, and a variety of factors influence its course.*

- The course of schizophrenia varies.
  - Some people have one or two episodes of psychosis and never have more (though this is rare).
  - Some have several months or years between episodes.
  - Others fluctuate rapidly between episodes of psychosis and periods of wellness.
- While the course is not predictable, there are skills that can protect against relapse such as
  - Consistently taking medication and consulting with your psychiatrist.
  - Consistent psychotherapy.
  - Social support from loved ones.
  - Consistent and sufficient sleep.
  - Maintaining low levels of stress.

## What Can the Family Do to Assist?

*Family members can also be helpful in protecting against an illness recurrence in a variety of ways.*

- Some ways in which the family can help include
    - Encouraging professional help-seeking and sticking to treatment (e.g., therapy and medication).
    - Noticing and helping identify new symptoms, changes in symptoms (e.g., frequency), and potential signs of relapse.
    - Learning the symptoms and understanding they are not the individual's fault.
    - Keeping a cohesive and warm environment in the home (avoiding criticism and hostility toward the person with a schizophrenia spectrum disorder).
    - Helping to maintain lower levels of stress both within the family environment and in their loved one by
        - Maintaining realistic expectations of their loved one and themselves (e.g., related to chores, school, work).
        - Encouraging a low-stress home environment (e.g., being less emotionally overinvolved and critical of their loved one).

---

*The content and format of this handout were inspired by Miklowitz and Goldstein (1997, p. 138).*

## Religion and Spirituality

*The following are questions to help guide discussion on religion and spirituality.*

### Religious/Spiritual Background

- In which religious tradition were you raised?
- Is religion or spirituality important to you?
- What do these terms mean to you?

### Current Religious/Spiritual Views

- What is your concept of God or a higher power?
- What is your main religious or spiritual identity?
- What effect does religion/spirituality have on you today?
- What is the role of prayer or meditation in your life?
- What is the primary content of your prayers or your main thoughts during meditation?
- What religious/spiritual beliefs and values are important to you? How are they applied in your daily life?
- What religious rituals and practices are important to you?
- Do your religious and spiritual beliefs influence the way you look at problems, such as mental illness, and the way you think about your health?
- What religious or spiritual issues, if any, have caused problems in your relationships?
- If resolved, how did you resolve them?

## Existential and Philosophical Beliefs

*The following are questions to help guide discussion on existential and philosophical beliefs.*

### Existential/Philosophical Background

- Were you raised in any spiritual tradition?
- What are your guiding existential or philosophical beliefs (e.g., Are human beings basically good or bad? What is the purpose or meaning of life?)
- Are there any supreme beings? What is your concept of a higher power?

### Current Existential/Philosophical Views

- Which of your values are most important to you?
- What are your ideas about morality and the concepts of right and wrong?
- Do you have any rituals or practices that are important to you (e.g., meditation, yoga)?
- Do your existential/philosophical beliefs influence the way you look at problems, such as mental illness, and the way you think about your health?
- Have any of your existential/philosophical beliefs caused problems in your relationships?
- If resolved, how did you resolve them?

## Spiritual Methods of Coping

*The following handout will be used to guide the discussion of spiritual/religious or philosophical/ existential beliefs, behaviors, and values thought to improve coping and mental and emotional well-being.*

### Develop Emotional Awareness

- Foster positive attitudes such as forgiveness, gratitude, and generosity (these are at the heart of most major world religions)
- Cultivate positive emotions such as love, empathy, and compassion
- Master and reduce toxic and painful emotions such as intense anger, fear, hatred, and resentment

### Develop a Calm Mind

- Practice prayer, yoga, contemplation, and/or meditation
- Take walks in nature
- Engage in spiritual/philosophical readings
- Participate at church, temple, mosque, or other organized groups
- Consult with priests, rabbis, imams, scholars, or other health healers for advice on managing illness or psychological distress
- Engage your values (e.g., giving back through volunteering)
- Engage in other soothing rituals (e.g., chanting or singing hymns, lighting incense or candles, aromatherapy)

**Handout 12**

## Communication and Culture

*Communication can be more effective when we try to be understanding of cultural norms.*

- Norms of communication vary by culture and sometimes even within cultures.
- Norms of communication can also vary based on gender, age, generation, and type of relationship (e.g., parent/child vs. siblings).
- Communication can be misinterpreted when we are unaware of the norms of the other person's culture.
- Note that the exercises provided in this module for effective communication are just guidelines. They may need to be modified for your particular needs based on your culture and the types of relationships among members of your family.

Here are some guiding questions to help you think about communication in your family.

In your culture and family,

1. Do you place a stronger value on direct or indirect patterns of communication?
2. How are communication difficulties raised and addressed?
3. Are there norms that dictate who (e.g., men, elders) and when different members should speak up or remain silent?
4. What areas are important to communicate about directly?
5. Are there topics or circumstances that are off limits for discussion?

*As noted on p. 19, the Communication Training Module was heavily influenced by earlier family treatments for schizophrenia (Falloon et al., 1984, pp. 207–260) and bipolar disorder (Goldstein & Miklowitz, 1997, pp. 187–214).*

## Expressing Positive Feelings

*The following handout is on expressing positive feelings.*

1. Be specific about what the person did that pleased you.
2. Say how that action made you feel.

Telling others specifically *what* they did and *how* it made you feel is more effective than making general statements of appreciation. This gives others a clearer sense of how to please you again in the future.

| Example | |
| --- | --- |
| How do these responses make you feel? Do you have a preference for one? Why? | |
| "Thanks for helping out today. You did a lot of hard work." | "I really appreciate that you pitched in and cleaned the bathrooms today. It made me feel like you care about our home, and that made me feel so grateful." |

*The content and format of this handout were inspired by Miklowitz and Goldstein (1997, p. 198) and by Falloon et al. (1984, p. 218).*

## Listening Attentively

*Effective communication lessens stress levels among those involved by reducing ambiguity, particularly when stressful situations could give rise to ineffective communication.*

1. Acknowledge the speaker.
   - Often this means looking directly at them or offering another form of appropriate eye contact.
2. Show you are interested by
   - Paraphrasing what the person has said.
   - Asking questions to help clarify misunderstandings, and show that you are paying attention.
   - Using exclamations, such as "uh-huh" or "I see."
   - Using nonverbal cues such as nodding your head, leaning in, or moving closer to the speaker.

| Example |
| --- |
| *Imagine you had a difficult day at work and want to convey this to a family member. You say, "Today was very stressful. My boss criticized me in front of my colleagues." How does each of these patterns of response make you feel? Do you have a preference for one? Why?* |

| While walking away from you, the listener says, "I had a difficult day too; maybe you should get another job." | While looking at you, the listener says, "Oh gosh, sounds like you had a really tough day. I'm sorry to hear that. What exactly did your boss say that upset you?" |
| --- | --- |

*The content and format of this handout were inspired by Miklowitz and Goldstein (1997, p. 203) and by Falloon et al. (1984, p. 231).*

## Making a Positive Request

*The following handout provides a guideline for how to make a positive request.*

Be specific and

1. Say exactly what you would like to happen.
2. Tell them how you think you would feel, if they complied with your request.

For example, you could say

1. I would really appreciate it if you (*did X thing*).
2. I think I would feel more (*feeling*).

| Example |
| --- |
| *Which one is more likely to get positive results? Why?* |

| | |
| --- | --- |
| "I would really appreciate it if in the future, you could tell me where you are going and when you will be back. Instead of feeling jumpy and anxious, I think I would feel much calmer, knowing that you were safe." | "You are so inconsiderate. You didn't even bother to tell me you were going out or when you would be back. You prefer to just let me stew and worry about you. You clearly don't care about my feelings." |

---

*The content and format of this handout were inspired by Miklowitz and Goldstein (1997, p. 209) and by Falloon et al. (1984, p. 223).*

## Expressing Specific Negative Feelings and Suggesting a Behavioral Change

*The following handout is largely about expressing negative feelings.*

### Expressing Negative Feelings

1. Say exactly what the person did that upset you.
2. Tell them how it made you feel.
3. Offer future direction.
4. Provide potential strategies that you and the person might do to help prevent similar events from happening in the future.

| Example |  |
| --- | --- |
| *Which response is most likely to get a positive result? Why?* |  |
| "Last night we had agreed to watch a program on TV together at 7. When you arrived late, it hurt my feelings. It made me feel like you don't respect my time and feelings. Moving forward, can we briefly discuss our daily plans in the morning, so we have a realistic timeframe for our evening plans?" | "I can't believe you got home late last night again, after we had agreed to watch a program on TV together at 7. You only care about yourself. You don't care about my plans. Next time, I'll start the show without you, because you clearly don't care anyway." |

*The content and format of this handout were inspired by Miklowitz and Goldstein (1997, p. 212) and by Falloon et al. (1984, p. 229).*

## Problem-Solving and Culture

*Effective problem solving is an important life skill. To hone problem-solving skills, it is helpful to begin by examining how you and your family and/or other groups in which you frequently interact typically solve problems. It is then useful to reflect on which of these strategies have been effective and which could be improved.*

- How do you typically solve problems? For example, do you generally turn to your faith? Do you tend to focus on one aspect of the problem, which may unintentionally cloud your view on other features of the problem?
- Are there "rules" in your family or culture that guide whether a problem should be talked about openly versus kept hidden?
- How do your values influence what is viewed as a major problem that *must* be solved directly versus a minor one that you may be willing to *let go of* or ignore altogether?

The following are some guiding questions to help you examine problem-solving in your family and culture:

1. How do you decide whether a problem is within or outside your control?
2. How do you decide what problems are or are not worth your time and energy?
3. How do you feel when you've solved a problem? Are there core features to your approach that lead to a successful resolution?
4. How do you feel when the problem you thought you had solved, remains a problem? What, if anything, do you do to follow up?

---

*As noted on p. 19, the Problem-Solving Module was heavily influenced by earlier family treatments for schizophrenia (Falloon et al., 1984, pp. 261–283) and bipolar disorder (Goldstein & Miklowitz, 1997, pp. 237–260).*

## Problem-Solving Overview

*This handout focuses on how to solve problems as a family. It is helpful to try out this strategy with a relatively simple problem first to learn the steps, before moving on to solving more complex problems.*

It is important to do these steps one by one, especially as you begin to learn this process.

1. Agree on the problem.
    - How do you decide on whether a problem is worthwhile to solve?
    - Problems may be things that make you feel stressed out or have been counterproductive.
    - Try to ensure you are accurately identifying the core problem, rather than a superficial one.
    - Do all members of the family view the problem in the same way?
2. Suggest several possible solutions.
    - Brainstorming "outside-the-box" solutions can also help generate ones that may be useful.
3. Discuss pros and cons and agree on the best solutions.
    - You may find that you care more about a particular pro than a con.
4. Plan and carry out the best solution(s).
    - This can be more than one solution or can incorporate parts of more than one solution.
5. Praise efforts and review effectiveness.
    - The result will likely not be perfect, but praising your effort, and the efforts of your family members, is important.

---

*The content and format of this handout were inspired by Miklowitz & Goldstein (1997, p. 241).*

**Handout 19**

## Guided Problem-Solving

*This handout presents a step-by-step guide to structure the problem-solving process.*

### Step 1

- Define the problem in your own words and describe why you think it is a problem. What family values or goals does this problem violate or interfere with?
- Use the communication skills you've learned to get everybody's input.

_____

_____

_____

### Step 2

As a family, brainstorm several possible solutions, including out-of-the-box ones. Do not evaluate (judge) any of the solutions at this stage.

1. _____
2. _____
3. _____
4. _____
5. _____
6. _____
7. _____

## Step 3

As a family, discuss each possible solution and list the advantages and disadvantages of each.

| Advantages | Disadvantages |
|---|---|
| 1 | 1 |
| 2 | 2 |
| 3 | 3 |
| 4 | 4 |
| 5 | 5 |
| 6 | 6 |
| 7 | 7 |

## Step 4

- Remind yourselves of the agreed upon problem and choose which solution, *or* solutions, you agree would work best to alleviate the problem?

_____

_____

_____

_____

## Step 5

- How will you carry out the chosen solution(s), *and* when will you do so?
- Make a plan.
  A. Who will do what? List.

  - _____
  - _____
  - _____
  - _____

  B. What will you need? How will you get what you need?

  - _____
  - _____
  - _____

C. Make another plan for things that might go wrong. Specifically, if things do go wrong, how will you move ahead?

    ■ _____

    ■ _____

    ■ _____

D. Implement the plan.

## Step 6

Review. Was everyone able to complete their part of the solution? How did it go?

_____

_____

_____

_____

## Step 7

If the problem is not resolved, go back to Step 1, and try to understand the problem better. Perhaps the problem needs to be broken into smaller, more easily solved, segments. Do not become discouraged and do try again.

_____

_____

_____

_____

*The content and format of this handout were inspired by Miklowitz and Goldstein (1997, pp. 248–249) and by Falloon et al. (1984, p. 263).*

# References

Acosta, F. (1982). Group therapy with Spanish-speaking patients. In R. Becerra, M. Karno, & J. Escobar (Eds.), *Mental health and Hispanic Americans: Clinical Perspectives* (pp. 183–197). New York, NY: Grune & Stratton.

Adames, H. Y., Chavez-Dueñas, N. Y., Sharma, S., & La Roche, M. J. (2018). Intersectionality in psychotherapy: The experiences of an AfroLatinx queer immigrant. *Psychotherapy*, *55*(1), 73–79. https://doi.org/10.1037/pst0000152

Agyemang, C., Bhopal, R., & Bruijnzeels, M. (2005). Negro, Black, Black African, African Caribbean, African American or what? Labelling African origin populations in the health arena in the 21st century. *Journal of Epidemiology & Community Health*, *59*(12), 1014–1018. https://dx.doi.org/10.1136/jech.2005.035964

Alba, R., Logan, J., Lutz, A., & Stults, B. (2002). Only English by the third generation? Loss and preservation of the mother tongue among the grandchildren of contemporary immigrants. *Demography*, *39*(3), 467–484. https://doi.org/10.1353/dem.2002.0023

Almeida, R. (2005). Asian Indian families. In M. McGoldrick, J. Giordano, & N. Garcia-Peto (Eds.), *Ethnicity and Family Therapy* (pp. 377–394). New York, NY: Guilford.

Ano, G. G., & Vasconcelles, E. B. (2005). Religious coping and psychological adjustment to stress: A meta-analysis. *Journal of Clinical Psychology*, *61*(4), 461–480. https://doi.org/10.1002/jclp.20049

Aponte, J. F., & Johnson, L. R. (2000). The impact of culture on the intervention and treatment of ethnic populations. In J. F. Aponte & J. Wohl (Eds.), *Psychological Intervention and Cultural Diversity* (pp. 18–39). Boston, MA: Allyn & Bacon.

Arieli, S., & Sagiv, L. (2018). Culture and problem-solving: Congruency between the cultural mindset of individualism versus collectivism and problem type. *Journal of Experimental Psychology: General*, *147*(6), 789–814. https://doi.org/10.1037/xge0000444

Ascher-Svanum, H., Faries, D. E., Zhu, B., Ernst, F. R., Swartz, M. S., & Swanson, J. W. (2006). Medication adherence and long-term functional outcomes in the treatment of schizophrenia in usual care. *Journal of Clinical Psychiatry, 67*(3), 453–460. https://doi.org/10.4088/JCP.v67n0317

Baier, M. (2010). Insight in schizophrenia: a review. *Current Psychiatry Reports, 12*(4), 356–361. https://doi.org/10.1007/s11920-010-0125-7

Barakat, H. (2004). The Arab family and the challenge of social transformation. In H. Moghissi (Ed.), *Women and Islam: Critical Concepts in Sociology* (Vol. 1, pp. 145–165). London, England: Taylor and Francis.

Barlow, D. H. (2004). Psychological treatments. *American Psychologist, 59*(9), 869–878.

Barlow, D. H. (2010). Negative effects from psychological treatments: A perspective. *American Psychologist, 65*(1), 13–20.

Barrio, C., Hernández, M., & Barragan, A. (2011). Serving Latino families caring for a person with serious mental illness. In L. Buki & L. M. Piedra (Eds.), *Creating Infrastructure for Latino Mental Health* (Vol. 1, pp. 159–175). New York, NY: Springer.

Barrio, C., & Yamada, A. M. (2010). Culturally based intervention development: The case of Latino families dealing with schizophrenia. *Research on Social Work Practice, 20*(5), 483–492. https://doi.org/10.1177/1049731510361613

Baskin, D. (1984). Cross cultural conceptions of mental illness. *Psychiatric Quarterly, 56*(1), 45–53. https://doi.org/10.1007/BF01324631

Berman, T. (2010). The ability to verbalize one's needs clearly in a geriatric population. In S. S. Fehr (Eds.), *101 Interventions in Group Therapy* (pp. 233–241). New York, NY: Routledge.

Berry, J. W. (2005). Acculturation: Living successfully in two cultures. *International Journal of Intercultural Relations, 29*(6), 697–712. https://doi.org/10.1016/j.ijintrel.2005.07.013

Berry, J. W. (2006). Acculturative stress. In P. T. P. Wong & L. C. J. Wong (Eds.), *Handbook of Multicultural Perspectives on Stress and Coping* (pp. 287–298). New York, NY: Springer.

Berry, J. W., & Sabatier, C. (2010). Acculturation, discrimination, and adaptation among second generation immigrant youth in Montreal and Paris. *International Journal of Intercultural Relations, 34*(3), 191–207. https://doi.org/10.1016/j.ijintrel.2009.11.007

Bhugra, D. (2005). The global prevalence of schizophrenia. *PLoS Medicine, 2*(5), E151. https://doi.org/10.1371/journal.pmed.0020151.g001

Bhugra, D., & McKenzie, K. (2003, September). Expressed emotion across cultures. *Advances in Psychiatric Treatment, 9*(5), 342–348. https://doi.org/10.1192/apt.9.5.342

Black, L., & Jackson, V. (2005). Families of African origin. In M. McGoldrick, J. Giordano, & N. Garcia-Preto (Eds.), *Ethnicity and family therapy* (3rd ed., pp. 77–152). New York, NY: Guilford Press.

Bono, G., McCullough, M. E., & Root, L. M. (2008). Forgiveness, feeling connected to others, and well-being: Two longitudinal studies. *Personality and Social Psychology Bulletin, 34*(2), 182–195. https://doi.org/10.1177/0146167207310025

Borelli, J. L., Sohn, L., Wang, B. A., Hong, K., DeCoste, C., & Suchman, N. E. (2019). Therapist–client language matching: Initial promise as a measure of therapist–client relationship quality. *Psychoanalytic Psychology, 36*(1), 9–18. https://doi.org/10.1037/pap0000177

Bowie, C. R., & Harvey, P. D. (2008). Communication abnormalities predict functional outcomes in chronic schizophrenia: differential associations with social and adaptive functions. *Schizophrenia Research, 103*(1–3), 240–247. https://doi.org/10.1016/j.schres.2008.05.006

Bradford, D., Stroup, S., & Liberman, J. (2002). Pharmacological treatments for schizophrenia. In P. E. Nathan & J. M. Gorman (Eds.), *A guide to treatments that work* (Vol. 2, pp. 169–200). Oxford, England: Oxford University Press.

Brown, C. A., & Weisman de Mamani, A. (2018). The mediating effect of family cohesion in reducing patient symptoms and family distress in a culturally informed family therapy for schizophrenia: A parallel-process latent-growth model. *Journal of Consulting and Clinical Psychology, 86*(1), 1–14. https://doi.org/10.1037/ccp0000257

Caqueo-Urizar, A., Urzúa, A., Boyer, L., & Williams, D. R. (2016). Religion involvement and quality of life in patients with schizophrenia in Latin America. *Social Psychiatry and Psychiatric Epidemiology, 51*(4), 521–528. https://doi.org/10.1007/s00127-015-1156-5

Cauce, A. M., & Domenech-Rodríguez, M. (2002). Latino families: Myths and realities. In J. M. Contreras, K. A. Kerns, & A. M. Neal-Barnett (Eds.), *Latino children and families in the United States: Current research and future directions* (pp. 3–25). Westport, CT: Praeger.

Chatters, L. M., Taylor, R. J., Jackson, J. S., & Lincoln, K. D. (2008). Religious coping among African Americans, Caribbean blacks and non-Hispanic Whites. *Journal of Community Psychology, 36*(3), 371–386. https://doi.org/10.1002/jcop.20202

Cheng, A. (2002). Expressed emotion: A cross-culturally valid concept? *British Journal of Psychiatry, 181*(6), 466–467. https://doi.org/10.1192/bjp.181.6.466

Chesley, N., & Fox, B. (2012). E-mail's use and perceived effect on family relationship quality: variations by gender and race/ethnicity. *Sociological Focus*, *45*(1), 63–84. https://doi.org/10.1080/00380237.2012.630906

Cohen, C. I., Jimenez, C., & Mittal, S. (2010). The role of religion in the well-being of older adults with schizophrenia. *Psychiatric Services*, *61*(9), 917–922. https://doi.org/10.1176/ps.2010.61.9.917.

Conoley, C. W., & Conoley, J. C. (2009). *Positive psychology and family therapy: creative techniques and practical tools for guiding change and enhancing growth*. Hoboken, NJ: Wiley.

Daley, D. C., & Marlatt, G. A. (2006). *Overcoming your alcohol or drug problem: Effective recovery strategies: Therapist guide* (2nd ed.). New York, NY: Oxford University Press.

Das, S., Punnoose, V. P., Doval, N., & Nair, V. Y. (2018). Spirituality, religiousness and coping in patients with schizophrenia: A cross sectional study in a tertiary care hospital. *Psychiatry Research*, *265*, 238–243. https://doi.org/10.1016/j.psychres.2018.04.030.

De Jong, G. F., & Madamba, A. B. (2001). A double disadvantage? Minority group, immigrant status, and underemployment in the United States. *Social Science Quarterly*, *82*(1), 117–130. https://doi.org/10.1111/0038-4941.00011

De Luca, S. M., & Escoto, E. R. (2012). The recruitment and support of Latino faculty for tenure and promotion. *Journal of Hispanic Higher Education*, *11*(1), 29–40. https://doi.org/10.1177/1538192711435552

Delgado-Romero, E. A., Manlove, A. N., Manlove, J. D., & Hernandez, C. A. (2006). Controversial issues in the recruitment and retention of Latino/a faculty. *Journal of Hispanic Higher Education*, *6*, 34–51. https://doi.org/10.1177/1538192706294903

Dickerson, F. B. (2004). Update on cognitive behavioral psychotherapy for schizophrenia: Review of recent studies. *Journal of Cognitive Psychotherapy: An International Quarterly*, *18*(3), 189–205. https://doi.org/10.1891/jcop.18.3.189.65654

Dillon, R. K., & McKenzie, N. J. (1998). The influence of ethnicity on listening, communication competence, approach, and avoidance. *International Journal of Listening*, *12*(1), 106–121. https://doi.org/10.1080/10904018.1998.10499021

Dingemanse, M., Roberts, S. G., Baranova, J., Blythe, J., Drew, P., Floyd, S., . . . Rossi, G. (2015). Universal principles in the repair of communication problems. *PloS One*, *10*(9), e0136100. https://doi.org/10.1371/journal.pone.0136100

Dixon, L. B., Dickerson, F., Bellack, A. S., Bennett, M., Dickinson, D., Goldberg, R. W., . . . Peer, J. (2010). The 2009 schizophrenia PORT psychosocial treatment recommendations and summary statements. *Schizophrenia Bulletin, 36*(1), 48–70.

Duan, C., Wei, M., & Wang, L. (2008). The role of individualism-collectivism in empathy: An exploratory study. *Asian Journal of Counselling, 15*(1), 57–81.

Emmons, R. A., & McCullough, M. E. (2003). Counting blessings versus burdens: an experimental investigation of gratitude and subjective well-being in daily life. *Journal of Personality and Social Psychology, 84*(2), 377–389.

Falloon, I. R., Boyd, J. L., & McGill, C. W. (1984). *Family care of schizophrenia: A problem-solving approach to the treatment of mental illness.* New York, NY: Guilford Press.

Friedman, M. L., Friedlander, M. L., & Blustein, D. L. (2005). Toward an Understanding of Jewish Identity: A Phenomenological Study. *Journal of Counseling Psychology, 52*(1), 77–83.

Gallup Poll. (n.d.). Do you believe in God? May 3–7, 2017. Retrieved from https://news.gallup.com/poll/1690/Religion.aspx

George, L. K., Larson, D. B., Koenig, H. G., & McCullough, M. E. (2000). Spirituality and health: What we know, what we need to know. *Journal of Social and Clinical Psychology, 19*(1), 102–116. https://doi.org/10.1521/jscp.2000.19.1.102

Giordano, J., & McGoldrick, M. (2005). Families of European Origin. In M. McGoldrick, J. Giordano, & N. Garcia-Preto (Eds.), *Ethnicity and family therapy* (3rd ed., pp. 501–519). New York, NY: Guilford Press.

Glenn, S. A. (2002). In the blood? Consent, descent, and the ironies of Jewish identity. *Jewish Social Studies, 8*(2/3), 139–152.

Goldstein, M. J., & Miklowitz, D. J. (1994). Family intervention for persons with bipolar disorder. In A. B. Hatfield (Ed.), *Family interventions in mental illness* (pp. 23–35). San Francisco, CA: Jossey-Bass.

Grover, S., Davuluri, T., & Chakrabarti, S. (2014). Religion, spirituality, and schizophrenia: A review. *Indian Journal of PSYCHOLOGICAL medicine, 36*(2), 119–124. https://doi.org/10.4103/0253-7176.130962

Gurak, K., & Weisman de Mamani, A. (2017). Caregiver expressed emotion and psychiatric symptoms in African-Americans with schizophrenia: An attempt to understand the paradoxical relationship. *Family Process, 56*, 476–486. https://doi.org/10.1111/famp.12188

Gurak, K. K., Weisman de Mamani, A., & Ironson, G. (2017). Does religiosity predict attrition from a culturally-informed family treatment for schizophrenia that targets religious coping?. *Journal of Consulting and Clinical Psychology, 85*(10), 937–949. https://doi.org/10.1037/ccp0000234

Güss, C. D., & Tuason, M. T. (2009). Fire and ice: Cultural influences on complex problem solving. In *Proceedings of the Annual Meeting of the Cognitive Science Society*, 31. Retrieved from https://escholarship.org/uc/item/194595pw

Gutiérrez-Maldonado, J., & Caqueo-Urízar, A. (2007). Effectiveness of a psycho-educational intervention for reducing burden in Latin American families of patients with schizophrenia. *Quality of Life Research*, *16*(5), 739–747. https://doi.org/10.1007/s11136-007-9173-9

Harrison, M. O., Koenig, H. G., Hays, J. C., Eme-Akwari, A. G., & Pargament, K. I. (2001). The epidemiology of religious coping: A review of recent literature. *International Review of Psychiatry*, *13*(2), 86–93. https://doi.org/10.1080/09540260124356

Hecht, M. L., & Faulkner, S. L. (2000). Sometimes Jewish, sometimes not: The closeting of Jewish American identity. *Communication Studies*, *51*(4), 372–387.

Heinke, M. S., & Louis, W. R. (2009). Cultural background and individualistic–collectivistic values in relation to similarity, perspective taking, and empathy. *Journal of Applied Social Psychology*, *39*(11), 2570–2590. https://doi.org/10.1111/j.1559-1816.2009.00538.x

Heresco-Levy, U., Greenberg, D., & Dasberg, H. (1990). Family expressed emotion: Concepts, dilemmas and the Israeli perspective. *Israel Journal of Psychiatry and Related Sciences*, *27*(4), 205–215.

Hines, P. M., & Boyd-Franklin, N. (2005). African American families. In M. McGoldrick, J. Giordano, & N. Garcia-Preto (Eds.), *Ethnicity and family therapy* (3rd ed., pp. 87–100). New York, NY: Guilford Press.

Humes, K., Jones, N. A., & Ramirez, R. R. (2011). *Overview of Race and Hispanic Origin: 2010*. Washington, DC: U.S. Census Bureau.

Institute of Medicine. (2001). *Crossing the quality chasm: A new health system for the 21st century*. Washington, DC: National Academy Press.

Institute of Medicine. (2015). *Psychosocial interventions for mental and substance use disorders: A framework for establishing evidence-based standards*. Washington, DC: National Academies Press.

Intersectionality. (n.d.). *Oxford's Lexico online dictionary*. Retrieved from https://www.lexico.com/en/definition/intersectionality

Jablensky, A., Sartorius, N., Ernberg, G., Anker, M., Korten, A., Cooper, J. E., & Bertelsen, A. (1992). Schizophrenia: Manifestations, incidence and course in different cultures. A World Health Organization ten-country study. *Psychological Medicine Monograph Supplement*, *20*, 1–97. https://doi.org/10.1017/s0264180100000904

Jenkins, J. H., Karno, M., de la Selva, A., & Santana, F. (1986). Expressed emotion in cross-cultural context: Familial responses to schizophrenic illness among Mexican Americans. In M. J. Goldstein, I. Hand, & K. Hahlweg (Eds.), *Treatment of schizophrenia* (pp. 35–49). Berlin, Germany: Springer. https://doi.org/10.1007/978-3-642-95496-2_4

Kempf-Leonard, K. (2007). Minority youths and juvenile justice: Disproportionate minority contact after nearly 20 years of reform efforts. *Youth Violence and Juvenile Justice*, 5(1), 71–87. https://doi.org/10.1177/1541204006295159

Kiang, L., Yip, T., Gonzales-Backen, M., Witkow, M., & Fuligni, A. J. (2006). Ethnic identity and the daily psychological well-being of adolescents from Mexican and Chinese backgrounds. *Child Development*, 77(5), 1338–1350. https://doi.org/10.1111/j.1467-8624.2006.00938.x

Kim, P. Y. (2017). Religious support mediates the racial microaggressions–mental health relation among Christian ethnic minority students. *Psychology of Religion and Spirituality*, 9(2), 148–157. https://doi.org/10.1037/rel0000076

Kingdon, D. G., & Turkington, D. (2005). *Cognitive therapy of schizophrenia*. New York, NY: Guilford.

Koenig, H. G. (2012). *Spirituality and health research: Methods, measurements, statistics, and resources*. West Conshohocken, PA: Templeton Foundation Press.

Koenig, H. G., Hays, J. C., George, L. K., Blazer, D. G., Larson, D. B., & Landerman, L. R. (1997). Modeling the cross-sectional relationships between religion, physical health, social support, and depressive symptoms. *American Journal of Geriatric Psychiatry*, 5(2), 131–144. https://doi.org/10.1097/00019442-199700520-00006

Koenig, H. G., Larson, D. B., & Weaver, A. J. (1998). Research on religion and serious mental illness. *New Directions for Mental Health Services*, 1998(80), 81–95. https://doi.org/10.1002/yd.23319988010

Kymalainen, J., & Weisman de Mamani, A. (2008). Expressed emotion, communication deviance and culture in families of patients with schizophrenia: A review of the literature. *Cultural Diversity and Ethnic Minority Psychology*, 14, 85–91. https://doi.org/10.1037/1099-9809.14.2.85

Kymalainen, J. A., Weisman, A. G., Rosales, G. A., & Armesto, J. C. (2006). Ethnicity, expressed emotion, and communication deviance in family members of patients with schizophrenia. *Journal of Nervous and Mental Disease*, 194, 391–396. https://doi.org/10.1097/01.nmd.0000221171.42027.5a

Latinos in America: A journey in stages. (2000, January 15). *Washington Post*. Retrieved from https://www.washingtonpost.com/wp-srv/WPcap/2000-01/16/078r-011600-idx.html

Lawless, J. L., & Pearson, K. (2008). The primary reason for women's underrepresentation? Reevaluating the conventional wisdom. *Journal of Politics*, *70*(1), 67–82. https://doi.org/10.1017/S002238160708005X

Le, A. T., & Miller, P. W. (2010). Glass ceiling and double disadvantage effects: Women in the US labour market. *Applied Economics*, *42*(5), 603–613. https://doi.org/10.1080/00036840701704501

Lebow, J. (2015). *Couple and family therapy: An integrative map of the territory*. Washington, DC: American Psychological Association.

Lee, E., & Mock, M. R. (2005). Asian families. In M. McGoldrick, J. Giordano, & N. Garcia-Preto (Eds.), *Ethnicity and family therapy* (3rd ed., pp. 269–289). New York, NY: Guilford Press.

Lefley, H. P. (1990). Culture and chronic mental illness. *Psychiatric Services*, *41*(3), 277–286. https://doi.org/10.1176/ps.41.3.277

Lehman, A. F., Lieberman, J. A., Dixon, L. B., McGlashan, T. H., Miller, A. L., Perkins, D. O., . . . Cook, I. (2004). Practice guideline for the treatment of patients with schizophrenia. *American Journal of Psychiatry*, *161*(2 Suppl.), 1–56.

Leong, F. T., & Lee, S. H. (2006). A cultural accommodation model for cross-cultural psychotherapy: Illustrated with the case of Asian Americans. *Psychotherapy: Theory, Research, Practice, Training*, *43*(4), 410–423. https://doi.org/10.1037/0033-3204.43.4.410

Leucht, S., Corves, C., Arbter, D., Engel, R. R., Li, C., & Davis, J. M. (2009). Second-generation versus first-generation antipsychotic drugs for schizophrenia: A meta-analysis. *The Lancet*, *373*(9657), 31–41. https://doi.org/10.1016/S0140-6736 (08)61764-X

Leung, P. K., & Boehnlein, J. K. (2005). Vietnamese families. In M. McGoldrick, J. Giordano, & N. Garcia-Preto (Eds.), *Ethnicity and family therapy* (3rd ed., pp. 363–373). New York, NY: Guilford Press.

Lincoln, K. D., Chatters, L. M., & Taylor, R. J. (2003). Psychological distress among Black and White Americans: Differential effects of social support, negative interaction and personal control. *Journal of Health and Social Behavior*, *44*(3), 390–407.

Linden, M., Pyrkosch, L., & Hundemer, H. P. (2008). Frequency and effects of psychosocial interventions additional to olanzapine treatment in routine care of schizophrenic patients. *Social Psychiatry and Psychiatric Epidemiology*, *43*(5), 373–379.

López, S. R., Nelson Hipke, K., Polo, A. J., Jenkins, J. H., Karno, M., Vaughn, C., & Snyder, K. S. (2004). Ethnicity, expressed emotion, attributions, and course of schizophrenia: Family warmth matters. *Journal of Abnormal Psychology*, *113*(3), 428–439. https://doi.org/10.1037/0021-843X.113.3.428

Lopez, S. R., Ramirez Garcia, J. I., Ullman, J. B., Kopelowicz, A., Jenkins, J., Breitborde, N. J. K., & Placencia, P. (2009). Cultural variability in the manifestation of expressed emotion. *Family Process, 48*(2), 179–194. https://doi.org/10.1111/j.1545-5300.2009.01276.x

Lucksted, A., McFarlane, W., Downing, D., & Dixon, L. (2012). Recent developments in family psychoeducation as an evidence-based practice. *Journal of Marital and Family Therapy, 38*(1), 101–121. https://doi.org/10.1111/j.1752-0606.2011.00256.x

Martinez de Andino, A., Brown, C., & Weisman de Mamani, A. (2018). Similaridades del terapeuta y paciente en factores socioculturales como predictores de la eficacia en una terapia para esquizofrenia informada por la cultura (pp. 285–304). In M. Valencia (Ed.), *Remisión y recuperación funcional: En depresión, trastorno bipolar y esquizofrenia* (APM Ediciones y Convenciones en Psiquiatría). Mexico City, Mexico.

Maura, J., & Weisman de Mamani, A. (2018). The feasibility of a culturally informed group therapy for patients with schizophrenia and their family members. *Psychotherapy, 55*(1), 27–38. https://doi.org/10.1037/pst0000109

McDermott, M., & Samson, F. L. (2005). White racial and ethnic identity in the United States. *Annual Review of Sociology, 31*, 245–261. https://doi.org/10.1146/annurev.soc.31.041304.122322

McHugh, R. K., & Barlow, D. H. (2010). Dissemination and implementation of evidence-based psychological interventions: A review of current efforts. *American Psychologist, 65*(2), 73–84.

Merrill, A. M., Karcher, N. R., Cicero, D. C., Becker, T. M., Docherty, A. R., & Kerns, J. G. (2017). Evidence that communication impairment in schizophrenia is associated with generalized poor task performance. *Psychiatry Research, 249*, 172–179. https://doi.org/10.1016/j.psychres.2016.12.051

Miklowitz, D. J., & Goldstein M. J. (1997). *Bipolar disorder: A family-focused treatment approach*. New York, NY: Guilford.

Mohr, S., Borras, L., Nolan, J., Gillieron, C., Brandt, P. Y., Eytan, A., . . . Koenig, H. G. (2012). Spirituality and religion in outpatients with schizophrenia: a multi-site comparative study of Switzerland, Canada, and the United States. *International Journal of Psychiatry in Medicine, 44*(1), 29–52. https://doi.org/10.2190/PM.44.1.c

Mohr, S., Brandt, P. Y., Borras, L., Gilliéron, C., & Huguelet, P. (2006). Toward an integration of spirituality and religiousness into the psychosocial dimension of schizophrenia. *American Journal of Psychiatry, 163*(11), 1952–1959.

Möller, H. J. (2007). Clinical evaluation of negative symptoms in schizophrenia. *European Psychiatry*, *22*(6), 380–386. https://doi.org/10.1016/j.eurpsy.2007.03.010

Mora, M. T., Villa, D. J., & Dávila, A. (2006). Language shift and maintenance among the children of immigrants in the US: Evidence in the Census for Spanish speakers and other language minorities. *Spanish in Context*, *3*(2), 239–254. https://doi.org/10.1075/sic.3.2.04mor

Moua, M. Y., & Lamborn, S. D. (2010). Hmong American adolescents' perception of ethnic socialization practices. *Journal of Adolescent Research*, *25*, 416–440. http://dx.doi.org/10.1177/0743558410361369

Nguyen, C. P., Wong, Y. J., Juang, L. P., & Park, I. J. (2015). Pathways among Asian Americans' family ethnic socialization, ethnic identity, and psychological well-being: A multigroup mediation model. *Asian American Journal of Psychology*, *6*(3), 273–280. https://doi.org/10.1037/aap0000026

Nobles, W. (2004). African philosophy: Foundations for Black psychology. In R. Jones (Ed.), *Black psychology* (4th ed., pp. 280–292). New York: Harper & Row.

Nolan, J. A., McEvoy, J. P., Koenig, H. G., Hooten, E. G., Whetten, K., & Pieper, C. F. (2012). Religious coping and quality of life among individuals living with schizophrenia. *Psychiatric Services*, *63*(10), 1051–1054. https://doi.org/10.1176/appi.ps.201000208.

O'Driscoll, C., Sener, S. B., Angmark, A., & Shaikh, M. (2019). Caregiving processes and expressed emotion in psychosis: A cross-cultural meta-analytic review. *Schizophrenia Research*, *208*, 8–15. https://doi.org/10.1016/j.schres.2019.03.020

Olivares, J. M., Sermon, J., Hemels, M., & Schreiner, A. (2013). Definitions and drivers of relapse in patients with schizophrenia: A systematic literature review. *Annals of General Psychiatry*, *12*(1), 32. https://doi.org/10.1186/1744-859X-12-32

Organista, K. C., & Muñoz, R. F. (1996). Cognitive behavioral therapy with Latinos. *Cognitive and Behavioral Practice*, *3*(2), 255–270. https://doi.org/10.1016/S1077-7229(96)80017-4

Pargament, K. I., Koenig, H. G., Tarakeshwar, N., & Hahn, J. (2004). Religious coping methods as predictors of psychological, physical and spiritual outcomes among medically ill elderly patients: A two-year longitudinal study. *Journal of Health Psychology*, *9*(6), 713–730. https://doi.org/10.1177/1359105304045366

Passel, J., Livingston, G., & Cohn, D. (2012, May 17). Explaining why minority births now outnumber white births. *PEW Research Center: Social & Demographic Trends*. Retrieved from https://www.

pewsocialtrends.org/2012/05/17/explaining-why-minority-births-now-outnumber-white-births/

Payne, I. R., Bergin, A. E., Bielema, K. A., & Jenkins, P. H. (1991). Review of religion and mental health: Prevention and the enhancement of psychosocial functioning. *Prevention in Human Services, 9*(2), 11–40. https://doi.org/10.1300/J293v09n02_02

Perivoliotis, D., Grant, P. M., Peters, E. R., Ison, R., Kuipers, E., & Beck, A. T. (2010). Cognitive insight predicts favorable outcome in cognitive behavioral therapy for psychosis. *Psychosis, 2*(1), 23–33. ttps://doi.org/10.1080/17522430903147520

PEW Research Center, Social & Demographic Trends. (2018, June 13). The age gap in religion across the world: 3. How religious commitment varies by country among people of all ages. Retrieved from https://www.pewforum.org/2018/06/13/how-religious-commitment-varies-by-country-among-people-of-all-ages/

Propst, L. R., Ostrom, R., Watkins, P., Dean, T., & Mashburn, D. (1992). Comparative efficacy of religious and nonreligious cognitive-behavioral therapy for the treatment of clinical depression in religious individuals. *Journal of Consulting and Clinical Psychology*, 60(1), 94–103.

Radhakrishnan, P., & Chan, D. K. S. (1997). Cultural differences in the relation between self-discrepancy and life satisfaction. *International Journal of Psychology, 32*(6), 387–398.

Roberts, D. L., Penn, D. L., & Combs, D. R. (2015*). Social cognition and interaction training (SCIT): Group psychotherapy for schizophrenia and other psychotic disorders, clinician guide.* New York, NY: Oxford University Press.

Robinson, J. H., & Fisher, A. (1992). The importance of a good kibun in the ESL classroom. *MinneTESOL Journal, 10*, 87–99.

Rodriguez, N., Mira, C. B., Paez, N. D., & Myers, H. F. (2007). Exploring the complexities of familism and acculturation: Central constructs for people of Mexican origin. *American Journal of Community Psychology, 39*(1–2), 61–77. https://doi.org/10.1007/s10464-007-9090-7

Rogan, R. G., & Hammer, M. R. (1998). An exploratory study of message affect behavior: A comparison between African Americans and Euro-Americans. *Journal of Language and Social Psychology, 17*(4), 449–464. https://doi.org/10.1177/0261927X980174002

Rosenfarb, I. S., Bellack, A. S., & Aziz, N. (2006). Family interactions and the course of schizophrenia in African American and White patients. *Journal of Abnormal Psychology, 115*(1), 112–120. https://doi.org/10.1037/0021-843X.115.1.112

Rosmarin, D. (2019, November). *Flexible spiritually integrated cognitive behavioral treatment for acute psychiatric care: A feasibility study among clinically & spiritually diverse patients.* Paper presented at the Association for Behavioral and Cognitive Therapies, Atlanta, GA.

Rosmarin, D. H., & Pirutinsky, S. (2020). Do religious patients need religious psychotherapists? A naturalistic treatment matching study among orthodox Jews. *Journal of Anxiety Disorders, 69*, 102170. https://doi.org/10.1016/j.janxdis.2019.102170

Sadath, A., Kumar, R., & Karlsson, M. (2018). Expressed emotion research in India: A narrative review. *Indian Journal of Psychological Medicine, 41*(1), 18–26. https://doi.org/10.4103/ijpsym.ijpsym_235_18

Saha, S., Chant, D., Welham, J., & McGrath, J. (2005). A systematic review of the prevalence of schizophrenia. *PLoS Medicine, 2*(5), e141. https://doi.org/10.1371/journal.pmed.0020141

Salinas, C. (2015). Understanding and meeting the needs of Latina/o students in higher education. In P. Sasso & J. Devitis (Eds.), *Today's college students* (pp. 21–37). New York, NY: Peter Lang.

Salinas, C., Jr., & Lozano, A. (2017). Mapping and recontextualizing the evolution of the term Latinx: An environmental scanning in higher education. *Journal of Latinos and Education, 18*(4), 302–315. https://doi.org/10.1080/15348431.2017.1390464

Sam, D. L., & Berry, J. W. (Eds.). (2006). *The Cambridge handbook of acculturation psychology.* Cambridge, England: Cambridge University Press.

Sanders, P. W., Allen, G. K., Fischer, L., Richards, P. S., Morgan, D. T., & Potts, R. W. (2015). Intrinsic religiousness and spirituality as predictors of mental health and positive psychological functioning in Latter-Day Saint adolescents and young adults. *Journal of Religion and Health, 54*(3), 871–887. https://doi.org/10.1007/s1094

Sedikides, C., Gaertner, L., & Toguchi, Y. (2003). Pancultural self-enhancement. *Journal of Personality and Social Psychology, 84*(1), 60–79. https://doi.org/10.1037/0022-3514.84.1.60

Segal, E. A., Gerdes, K. E., Mullins, J., Wagaman, M. A., & Androff, D. (2011). Social empathy attitudes: Do Latino students have more? *Journal of Human Behavior in the Social Environment, 21*(4), 438–454. https://doi.org/10.1080/10911359.2011.566445

Sharif, Z., Bradford, D., Stroup, S., & Lieberman, J. (2007). Pharmacological treatment of schizophrenia. In P. E. Nathan & J. M. Gorman (Eds.), *A guide to treatments that work* (4th ed., pp. 203–242). Oxford, England: Oxford University Press.

Singelis, T. M. (1994). The measurement of independent and interdependent self-construals. *Personality and Social Psychology Bulletin, 20*(5), 580–591. https://doi.org/10.1177/0146167294205014

Singer, M. T., & Wynne, L. C. (1965). Thought disorder and family relations of schizophrenics: IV. Results and implications. *Archives of General Psychiatry, 12*(2), 201–212.

Singh, S. P., Harley, K., & Suhail, K. (2013). Cultural specificity of emotional overinvolvement: A systematic review. *Schizophrenia Bulletin, 39*(2), 449–463. https://doi.org/10.1093/schbul/sbr170.

Sokol, L., & Fox, M. (2019). *The comprehensive clinician's guide to cognitive behavioral therapy.* Eau Claire, WI: PESI.

Soliz, J., Thorson, A. R., & Rittenour, C. E. (2009). Communicative correlates of satisfaction, family identity, and group salience in multiracial/ethnic families. *Journal of Marriage and Family, 71*(4), 819–832. https://doi.org/10.1111/j.1741-3737.2009.00637.x

Speed, B. C., Goldstein, B. L., & Goldfried, M. R. (2018). Assertiveness training: A forgotten evidence-based treatment. *Clinical Psychology: Science and Practice, 25*(1), e12216. https://doi.org/10.1111/cpsp.12216

Suarez-Orozco, M., & Páez, M. (Eds.). (2002). *Latinos: Remaking America.* Berkeley, CA: University of California Press.

Swartz, M. S., Wagner, H. R., Swanson, J. W., Stroup, T. S., McEvoy, J. P., Canive, J. M., . . . Van Dorn, R. (2006). Substance use in persons with schizophrenia: Baseline prevalence and correlates from the NIMH CATIE study. *Journal of Nervous and Mental Disease, 194*(3), 164–172. https://doi.org/0.1097/01.nmd.0000202575.79453.6e

Szapocznik, J., & Kurtines, W. M. (1993). Family psychology and cultural diversity: Opportunities for theory, research, and application. *American Psychologist, 48*(4), 400–407.

Tandon, R., Gaebel, W., Barch, D. M., Bustillo, J., Gur, R. E., Heckers, S., . . . Carpenter, W. (2013). Definition and description of schizophrenia in the DSM-5. *Schizophrenia Research, 150*(1), 3–10. https://doi.org/10.1016/j.schres.2013.05.028

Telles, C., Karno, M., Mintz, J., Paz, G., Arias, M., Tucker, D., & Lopez, S. (1995). Immigrant families coping with schizophrenia behavioural family intervention v. case management with a low-income spanish-speaking population. *British Journal of Psychiatry, 167*(4), 473–479. https://doi.org/10.1192/bjp.167.4.473

Telzer, E. H., Masten, C. L., Berkman, E. T., Lieberman, M. D., & Fuligni, A. J. (2010). Gaining while giving: An fMRI study of the rewards of family assistance among White and Latino youth. *Social Neuroscience*, *5*(5–6), 508–518. https://doi.org/10.1080/17470911003687913

Thomason, T. (2012). Recommendations for counseling Native Americans: Results of a survey. *Journal of Indigenous Research*, *1*(2), 4.

Torrey, E. F. (1995). *Surviving schizophrenia: A Manual for families, consumers, and providers* (3rd ed.). New York, NY: Harper Perennial.

Triandis, H. C. (2001). Individualism and collectivism: Past, present, and future. In D. Matsumoto (Ed.), *The handbook of culture and psychology* (pp. 35–50). New York, NY: Oxford University Press.

Triandis, H. C. (2018). *Individualism and collectivism*. London, England: Routledge. (Original work published 1995)

Turcios-Cotto, V. Y., & Milan, S. (2013). Racial/ethnic differences in the educational expectations of adolescents: Does pursuing higher education mean something different to Latino students compared to White and Black students? *Journal of youth and adolescence*, *42*(9), 1399–1412. https://doi.org/10.1007/s10964-012-9845-9

U.S. Census Bureau. (2011). Overview of race and Hispanic origin: 2010. Retrieved from https://www.census.gov/prod/cen2010/briefs/c2010br-02.pdf

Valencia, M., Fresan, A., Juárez, F., Escamilla, R., & Saracco, R. (2013). The beneficial effects of combining pharmacological and psychosocial treatment on remission and functional outcome in outpatients with schizophrenia. *Journal of Psychiatric Research*, *47*(12), 1886–1892. https://doi.org/10.1016/j.jpsychires.2013.09.006

Van Gundy, K. T., Howerton-Orcutt, A., & Mills, M. L. (2015). Race, coping style, and substance use disorder among non-Hispanic African American and White young adults in South Florida. *Substance Use & Misuse*, *50*(11), 1459–1469. https://doi.org/10.3109/10826084.2015.1018544

Ventura, J., Lukoff, D., Nuechterlein, K. H., Liberman, R. P., Green, M. F., & Shaner, A. (1993). Brief Psychiatric Rating Scale (BPRS) expanded version: Scales, anchor points, and administration book. *International Journal of Methods in Psychiatric Research*, *3*, 227–243.

Vogt Yuan, A. S. (2010). Black–White differences in aging out of substance use and abuse. *Sociological Spectrum*, *31*(1), 3–31.

Walker, E., Kestler, L., Bollini, A., & Hochman, K. M. (2004). Schizophrenia: Etiology and course. *Annual Review of Psychology*, *55*, 401–430. https://doi.org/10.1146/annurev.psych.55.090902.141950

Watkins, P. C., Uhder, J., & Pichinevskiy, S. (2015). Grateful recounting enhances subjective well-being: The importance of grateful processing.

*Journal of Positive Psychology, 10*(2), 91–98. https://doi.org/10.1080/
17439760.2014.927909

Weintraub, M. J., Hall, D. L., Carbonella, J. Y., Weisman de Mamani, A.,
& Hooley, J. M. (2016). Integrity of literature on expressed emotion
and relapse in patients with schizophrenia verified by a p-curve analysis.
*Family Process, 56*(2), 436–444. https://doi.org/10.1111/famp.12208

Weisman, A. (1997). Understanding cross-cultural prognostic variability
for schizophrenia. *Cultural Diversity and Mental Health, 3*(1), 23–35.
https://doi.org/10.1037/1099-9809.3.1.23

Weisman, A., Gomes, L. G., & López, S. R. (2003). Shifting blame away
from ill relatives: Latino families' reactions to schizophrenia. *Journal of
Nervous and Mental Disease, 191*(9), 574–581. https://doi.org/10.1097/
01.nmd.0000087183.90174.a8

Weisman, A., & López, S. R. (1997). An attributional analysis of emotional
reactions to schizophrenia in Mexican and Anglo-American cultures.
*Journal of Applied Social Psychology, 27*(3), 223–244. https://doi.org/
10.1111/j.1559-1816.1997.tb00630.x

Weisman, A. G., Rosales, G., Kymalainen, J., & Armesto, J. (2005).
Ethnicity, family cohesion, religiosity and general emotional distress in patients with schizophrenia and their relatives. *Journal of
Nervous and Mental Disease, 193*, 359–368. https://doi.org/10.1097/
01.nmd.0000165087.20440.d1

Weisman de Mamani, A., Altamirano, O., McLaughlin, M., & Lopez,
D. (2020). Culture and family-based intervention for severe mental
health illness. In F. van de Vijver & W. K. Halford (Eds.), *Culture and
families: Research and practice*. New York, NY: Academic Press.

Weisman de Mamani, A., Gurak, K., & Suro, G. (2014). Serious mental
illness. In F. T. L. Leong (Ed.), *APA handbook of multicultural psychology*
(Vol. 2, pp. 345–359). Washington, DC: American Psychological
Association.

Weisman de Mamani, A. G., Kymalainen, J. A., Rosales, G. A., & Armesto,
J. C. (2007). Expressed emotion and interdependence in White and
Latino/Hispanic family members of patients with schizophrenia.
*Psychiatry Research, 151*(1–2), 107–113. https://doi.org/10.1016/
j.psychres.2006.11.007

Weisman de Mamani, A., & Suro, G. (2016). The effect of a culturally informed therapy on self-conscious emotions and burden in caregivers of
patients with schizophrenia: A randomized clinical trial. *Psychotherapy,
53*(1), 57–67. https://doi.org/10.1037/pst0000038

Weisman de Mamani, A. G., Tuchman, N., & Duarte, E. (2010).
Incorporating religion/spirituality into treatment for serious mental

illness. *Cognitive and Behavioral Practice, 17*(4), 348–357. https://doi. org/10.1016/j.cbpra.2009.05.003

Weisman de Mamani, A., Weintraub, M. J., Gurak, K., & Maura, J. (2014). A randomized clinical trial to test the efficacy of a family-focused, culturally informed therapy for schizophrenia. *Journal of Family Psychology, 28*(6), 800–810.

Weisman de Mamani, A., Weintraub, M. J., Maura, J., Martinez de Andino, A., Brown, C., & Gurak, K. (2017). Acculturation styles and their associations with psychiatric symptoms and quality of life in ethnic minorities with schizophrenia, *Psychiatry Research, 255*, 418–423. https://doi.org/10.1016/j.psychres.2017.06.074

Weisskirch, R. S., Kim, S. Y., Schwartz, S. J., & Whitbourne, S. K. (2016). The complexity of ethnic identity among Jewish American emerging adults. *Identity, 16*(3), 127–141.

White, G. M., & Marsella A. J. (1982). Introduction: Cultural conceptions in mental health research and practice. In A. J. Marsella & G. M. White (Eds.), *Cultural conceptions of mental health and therapy. culture, illness, and healing* (Vol. 4). Dordrecht, The Netherlands: Springer.

Wüsten, C., & Lincoln, T. M. (2017). The association of family functioning and psychosis proneness in five countries that differ in cultural values and family structures. *Psychiatry Research, 253*, 158–164. https://doi. org/10.1016/j.psychres.2017.03.041

Zangrilli, A., Ducci, G., Bandinelli, P. L., Dooley, J., McCabe, R., & Priebe, S. (2014). How do psychiatrists address delusions in first meetings in acute care? A qualitative study. *BMC Psychiatry, 14*(1), 178. https://doi. org/10.1186/1471-244X-14-178

Zha, P., Walczyk, J. J., Griffith-Ross, D. A., Tobacyk, J. J., & Walczyk, D. F. (2006). The impact of culture and individualism–collectivism on the creative potential and achievement of American and Chinese adults. *Creativity Research Journal, 18*(3), 355–366. https://doi.org/10.1207/ s15326934crj1803_10

Zinnbauer, B. J., & Pargament, K. I. (2005). Religiousness and spirituality. In R. F. Paloutzian & C. L. Park (Eds.), *Handbook of the psychology of religion and spirituality* (pp. 21–42). New York, NY: Guilford Press.